Art and Psychoanalysis

This book explores the concept of estrangement from a psychoanalytic perspective, intertwining art and aesthetics to offer a paradigm of the aesthetic experience.

Gabriela Goldstein suggests that an unexpected encounter with a work of art may lead to a state of poetic estrangement, promoting a possible reorganization of its subject's psychic economy. The conceptual work is illuminated with vignettes exploring the experience of this state of estrangement, reflecting on the encounter between the subject and the other/Other, between analyst and patient, and in the framework provided by the analytical situation. Finally, Goldstein considers how the metapsychology of aesthetic experience and its research contribute to clinical understanding of processes of deficient symbolization.

Art and Psychoanalysis will be key reading for psychoanalysts, artists, researchers, and teachers of art and psychoanalysis. It will also be of great interest to art therapists, students of art and the humanities, as well as other readers interested in an in-depth understanding of the aesthetic experience and creative processes.

Gabriela Goldstein, PhD, is a training analyst of International Psychoanalytical Association and FEPAL, and the former president of the Argentine Psychoanalytic Association. She is the author of several books including *Art in Psychoanalysis* and an architect and painter.

The International Psychoanalytical Association Current Challenges in Psychoanalysis Series
Series Editor: Silvia Flechner

Recent titles in the Series include

Psychoanalysis and Severe Disorders in Young Children
Clinical and Community Work with Autism Spectrum Disorder and Child Mental Health
Nahir Bonifacino

Couple Work, Work with Couples
Éric Smadja

Art and Psychoanalysis
Between the Dialectics of the Other and Poetic Estrangement
Gabriela Goldstein

'*Art and Psychoanalysis* is a brilliant and deeply reflective work by Dr. Gabriela Goldstein, where creativity and the unconscious engage in a powerful and illuminating dialogue. Drawing on her unique experience as a psychoanalyst, architect, and artist, Goldstein offers an original and sensitive exploration of aesthetic experience as a transformative event.

The book presents an articulate and rigorous exploration of the aesthetic encounter, weaving together theoretical concepts and clinical experience. Goldstein interlaces Freud's ideas on the unconscious and the uncanny, Winnicott's theories on transitional space and creativity, and Lacan's reflections on aesthetics, within a rich interdisciplinary framework.

One of the most compelling threads in the book is the development of poetic estrangement—understood as a new form of sensibility and thought—which reveals the transfiguring power of both aesthetic experience and psychoanalysis. This concept is tightly linked to the dialectic of the Other, which permeates both the creative process and the encounter with the artwork, opening a space where the aesthetic becomes inherently ethical.

For Goldstein, the aesthetic experience is not passive contemplation, but an affective, mobilizing, and potentially transformative event that calls the subject to a reconfiguration of their internal reality and their bond with others—and with Otherness.

This is a key book for psychoanalysts, scholars in the humanities, educators, and all those interested in the intersection of psychoanalysis and art. It invites readers into a transformative encounter—with art, with the unconscious, and with the eros of the psyche.

Reading it is a journey—one that reveals, page after page, surprise, pleasure, and a profound encounter with the deepest layers of oneself.'

Dr Carlos Weisse, *Training analyst, Asociacion Psicoanalítica Argentina (International Psychoanalytical Association, FEPAL), Writer, and Faculty, AEAPG*

Art and Psychoanalysis

Between the Dialectics of the Other and Poetic Estrangement

Gabriela Goldstein

Routledge
Taylor & Francis Group
LONDON AND NEW YORK

Designed cover image: Getty Images

First published 2026
by Routledge
4 Park Square, Milton Park, Abingdon, Oxon OX14 4RN

and by Routledge
605 Third Avenue, New York, NY 10158

Routledge is an imprint of the Taylor & Francis Group, an informa business

British Library Cataloguing-in-Publication Data
A catalogue record for this book is available from the British Library

ISBN: 978-1-032-96978-7 (hbk)
ISBN: 978-1-032-96976-3 (pbk)
ISBN: 978-1-003-59155-9 (ebk)

DOI: 10.4324/9781003591559

Typeset in Palatino
by KnowledgeWorks Global Ltd.

Contents

Acknowledgments

My gratitude to the institutions where I have presented over the years the productions and writings that shape this book, a new work. The central idea of this book was also the subject of my doctoral thesis, "A poetic estrangement", which explores the perspectives of art and psychoanalysis on the aesthetic experience. I defended my PhD thesis at the Universidad del Salvador (USAL) in 2016 and received cum laude approval with recommendation for publication. Previously, my book *La experiencia estética*, published in 2005 by Del Estante publishing house, served as an inspirational text for this research. This book is the result of many years of research on this topic. I express my gratitude to the symposiums on psychoanalysis and art of the IPA in Florence, in which I participated as a presenter and commentator and which stimulated enriching encounters. In them emerged the theme of narcissism and the effect of disencapsulation by art, which today is part of this book. I thank the APA, the Argentinian Psychoanalytic Association where I was trained, for opening the plurality of psychoanalytical ideas that bring links between art, aesthetics, psychoanalysis, and the clinic.

Thanks to Lucas Fragasso, my professor of aesthetics classes for more than 15 years who, together with my trajectory as a painter and architect, are an essential part of the aesthetic and creative experience that I conceptualize in these writings. I also thank my painter friends for the exchanges I have had with them. I also thank my painter friends for the exchanges and reflections. Thanks to my colleagues of the APA and the Latin American Board of Thinking on Winnicott, where I also presented writings on creativity and psychoanalysis. My recognitions to the APA group on art and psychoanalysis that I have been coordinating for years, as well as to my colleagues Carlos Weisse, Adolfo Benjamin, Jaime Szpilka, Jorge Kury, Leonor Valenti, and Norberto Marucco. I offer my gratitude to my teachers, both in painting and psychoanalysis.

I thank Silvia Acosta, always attentive to method and writing; Susan Rogers who overviews with love; Ale Marucco, whose brilliant clarity always accompanies me; and Patty Latosinski, dear friend who also supports me with lucidity and affection. Thanks to Belén and all the Busquet family, for all.

Special thanks to my parents for the freedom to think and choose, for their modernity, courage and generosity. Thank you, Raquel and Néstor (†). To Gabriel, my life partner, who encourages me in challenges and projects. To the loves of my life, Isabel and Lola, the most brilliant women I know, always attentive with ideas and affection. To Alejo and Immanuel, who reflect with us, and to the wonder of creation: Lorenzo, Raphael and Lucinda. I Thank you all.

G. Goldstein

Foreword

The International Psychoanalytic Association Publications Committee is honored to present a new book from the Current Challenges in Psychoanalysis series. This series delves into the evolving landscape of psychoanalytic practice, addressing contemporary issues such as trauma, cultural diversity, technology's influence, and shifts in psychoanalytical dynamics. Each volume offers concise, interdisciplinary insights from leading experts, bridging classical psychoanalytic theory with modern challenges. Designed for clinicians and researchers, this series is a vital resource for those seeking to navigate and innovate within today's complex therapeutic environment.

The IPA Publications Committee is pleased to publish Dr. Gabriela Goldstein's new book "Poetic Estrangement: Dialectics of the Other Between Art and Psychoanalysis".

This book presents the phenomenon of the encounter "between" subject and object like a dialectic, promoting a creative subjective dimension. This encounter is explored from the perspective of the relationship between psychoanalysis and art and provides theoretical and clinical research that, from the aesthetics of the encounter with art, reflects on the theoretical and clinical value of analytical thinking to understand the subjective impact of the aesthetic experience and creative processes itself.

The author delves into estrangement from a psychoanalytic perspective, intertwining art and aesthetics to propose a new paradigm for understanding aesthetic experience. Beginning with the notion of an "Aesthetics of the Encounter"—a dialectic of the Other between art and psychoanalysis—the author states that the aesthetic experience involves a meeting of the subject with the art object, characterized by an event that brings about a non-pathological form of estrangement, intimately tied to creative processes.

Goldstein also states that art has always been a subject of interest and has occupied, and still occupies, a preeminent place in life and psychoanalysis. In Chapter Two, the author explores the epistemological foundation for understanding the psychic dialectic through aesthetic terms, grounded in psychoanalysis. It examines how fantasy, symbolization, and poiesis serve as conditions for knowledge and creativity as core psychic functions. By investigating the transitional and creative aspects of estrangement, working through, and the "zone" of estrangement, the chapter offers a conceptualization of a metapsychology of estrangement, updating the dialectic of ineffable and surprising encounters that promote symbolization, mainly through the introduction of Eros into this experience.

The book also delves into the concept of estrangement, stating that estrangement is characterized by a sensation of unreality outside of pathology, akin to being in a dream. This aligns with Winnicott's concept of the "area of illusion," a state of bewilderment during the encounter that simultaneously elicits forms of pleasure specific to aesthetic experiences. She also explores the destinies and estrangement in hysteria and the disturbed signification of the body, focusing on key concepts such as the scopic drive, the role of language, narcissism, the unstable Other, decapsularization, regarding narcissism and melancholia, alongside the failed aestheticization of the self. It examines the link between aesthetics, estrangement, and art from a psychoanalytic metapsychological perspective, regarding the development of narcissism and the drives.

Goldstein also explores the approach to a psychoanalytic perspective in art as a possibility of psychic elaboration and the role of sublimation and "psychic work" relating art and creativity. This experience occurs in a between-space, transitional, movement characterized by a sublimation that reveals intertwined intrapsychic processes, related to perception. In this regard, she exposes how the image appears in art, something uncanny within the beauty, like a residue of the old narcissism, and the two aspects of it: Eros, life, pleasure, and the uncanny. In "aesthetic effect," the ominous condition and a limit to beauty must be present in the form of absence; it must be veiled.

This book will be an essential tool for psychoanalysts and therapists concerned with the value of art experiences and their impact on subjectivity, as well as artists involved with the subjective implications of the encounter between the subject and the art object.

The publication's committee is interested in sharing this new book with the psychoanalytic community and other related disciplines to expand their knowledge and acquaint them with the author.

Silvia Flechner
Series Editor
Chair IPA Publications Committee

Introduction

0.1 Freud on the Acropolis and the aesthetic experience

This book explores the concept of *estrangement* from a psychoanalytic perspective, intertwined with art and aesthetics to offer a paradigm of aesthetic experience, in principle, with art. Starting from the idea of an "aesthetics of the encounter": dialectics of the Other between Art and Psychoanalysis we propose that the aesthetic experience is an encounter of the subject with the art object with the character of an event that implies a form of non-pathological *estrangement* that includes creative processes. The encounter "between" subject and object implies a dialectic that from the phenomenon of estrangement promotes a poetic, creative dimension.

This book presents this phenomenon from the perspective of the relationship between psychoanalysis and art and provides a theoretical and clinical research that from the aesthetics of the encounter with art, as well as the aesthetic value of analytical work as the aesthetic experience, creates something new.

The notion of estrangement comes from Freud's strange experience in the Acropolis (Freud, 1936), when the "unusual phenomenon" that he defines as estrangement, beyond interpretations, is also conceived as part of an aesthetic experience (Goldstein, 2005), in the instant in which the encounter with the Acropolis becomes an encounter with the strange. The estrangement implies a state of unreality in relation to what is perceived, in which the boundaries between fantasy and reality are blurred, but at the margin of pathology.

In the letter "A disturbance of memory in the Acropolis", letter to Romain Rolland that Freud writes to him (1936, p. 209) on the occasion of his birthday, he relates an "unusual and enigmatic phenomenon" that happens to him in Athens. In front of the Acropolis, the "feeling of estrangement" that he says he had, precipitates some effects and questions that, beyond its interpretation, show that an aesthetic experience also takes place there. I find that in the Acropolis a sequence begins: in the *passage* from the small experience to alienation, a *space of experience* is revealed which, in the conditions in which this passage takes place, assumes the institution of aesthetic experience.

DOI: 10.4324/9781003591559-1

0.2 The story in Athens: Key to the aesthetic experience

In the manner of a fairy tale, Freud recounts in a dizzying tone his trip to Athens. He and his brother Alexander, ten years younger (curiously like Romain Rolland), undertook every year a vacation trip to the Mediterranean area for several weeks. On his brother's business they decided to go to Corfu, and unexpectedly at the insistence of a friend, they changed course for Athens, and despite Freud's astonishment, since they were both in a bad mood and saw nothing but impediments to the possibility of such a trip, they bought tickets for the Lloyd's ship to Greece. "It was very strange behavior," Freud admits. On arriving in Athens, he describes his unexpected impression and says: "On the evening of our arrival, I was standing on the Acropolis and gazing out over the landscape when suddenly this astonishing thought came to me: 'Then all this really exists just as we learned it at school! More accurately described: the person who made the utterance separated himself, more noticeably and sharply than ordinarily, from another who perceived that utterance, and both were astonished, though not at the same thing. One behaved as if under the impression of an indubitable observation he was compelled to believe in something whose reality had hitherto seemed uncertain. With slight exaggeration: it is as if someone, walking along Loch Ness in Scotland, suddenly saw the body of the much-mentioned monster slithering on the ground and was forced to admit: "So there is indeed this snake in the lake that I did not believe in!". Now the other person was astonished, and rightly so, for he had never known that the real existence of Athens, the Acropolis and that landscape had ever been doubted. He had rather expected a proverbial rapture and exaltation (Freud, 1936, p. 214).

What prevented Freud from affirmatively accepting the rapture in front of the Acropolis and enunciating the expected utterance of rapture? What led him to such a situation of living as two people, one giving an account of what he perceived, the other, bluntly showing his incredulity? What motions were awakened in him that led him to be estranged—as he himself describes it—and to split, *admitting at the same time the inadmissibility of this split*?

Freud's analysis of what he experienced at the Acropolis is based on the field of Oedipus and guilt, and although in agreement with his interpretation, I propose another approach, in which I believe I can demonstrate that the strangeness of his experience turns out to be what introduces the aesthetic experience.

0.3 Freud's interpretation

Freud undertakes the analysis of his experience, along the lines of the Oedipus: repression, guilt, overcoming the father and the superego. However, there are some questions that, in my opinion, go beyond this analysis. The feeling of alienation invites further inquiry. Something else happens that shocks Freud so much that he prefers not to elucidate. The fantasy that altered the memory, according to Freud, was that as a child at school, he did not believe in the existence of the Acropolis .... Therefore, we can understand the violent dazzled exclamation: "Then all this does indeed exist just as we learned it at school!" But the analysis of successive transfers in time and space in the labyrinths of his memory, discover the cause of his concealment: "to get there someday", and thus interprets the guilt of overcoming the father and the fear of success. It would then be a pitying motion, says Freud and gives an account of the sequence of events at the crossroads of his personal history, which contributes to support the theoretical edifice of psychoanalysis. Freud develops in this writing encounter three fundamental axes:

First, the feeling of guilt and "those who fail to succeed", both on the conceptual axis Oedipus-repression, guilt and parricide. This is the central path Freud chooses to delimit the field of analysis of the "little experience".

Then, the question of the self and defense mechanisms appears, a subject that Anna—his daughter—deals with in her book.

And, finally, the problem of the feeling of estrangement, a subject that opens spaces in disturbing areas, and Freud decides to "forbid himself to continue elucidating".

Where Freud stops, I propose to continue investigating, since *the event at the Acropolis allows us to continue thinking about the strange and the* Spaltung, *where another reading of the feeling of estrangement will be a revealing question of the aesthetic experience.* This is called a "feeling of alienation" (*Entfremdungsgefühl*), Freud says, "I tried to defend myself against it, and I succeeded at the cost of a false statement about the past" (1936, p. 218). He then determines that these are misunderstood phenomena, "unusual phenomena" that serve the defense, they want to keep something painful from the past away from the ego and to disprove it because it could cause pain, something repressed from the "mnemic treasure of the ego" says Freud (p. 219).

Now, if we start from the hypothesis that Freud, "enraptured" before the Acropolis, "loses himself" (Freud, 1927, p. 25), lets himself go, is alienated in what can be an aesthetic experience and is disturbed in such a way, we can think that something prevents him from being so intensely moved. In this way Freud accounts for a certain personal condition that he applies to the object of aesthetic experience. He needs to understand why certain works "*subject*" him to "such violent impressions", and admits that: "works of art, however, exert a powerful influence on me", he says before Michelangelo's *Moses* and confesses that he had to remain before them for hours, in order to "... apprehend *in my own way, that is, by reducing to concepts, that through which they worked on me in this way. When I cannot do this*", he states "... *I am almost incapable of obtaining any enjoyment whatsoever.*[1] A rationalistic or perhaps analytic disposition rebels in me so that I do not let myself be moved without knowing why I am moved, and what moves me" (Freud, 1914, p. 217).

In Athens, Freud could not remain for a long time studying the object of his experience as he did before the *Moses* in Rome, where he visited the work for three long weeks, and remained in front of the "choleric" statue, measuring it, observing it, and holding "its scornful gaze" (p. 219). But on the Acropolis of Athens, he had neither time nor physical nor intellectual distance to "analyze." He could not approach the object of art cautiously, and with surprise the aesthetic experience happened to him without time to set conceptual barriers, and he was surprised and split in the face of this dangerous encounter. However, in this way, he assumed a necessary risk, the risk implied by the condition that art imposes on us in the aesthetic experience.

0.4 From aesthetics

Starting from conceptualizations coming from modern art and Aesthetics, I suggest some questions regarding the aesthetic experience today, whose main characteristic is the configuration of a "disturbing region"—as Agamben (1995), a contemporary philosopher who speaks about a place without men or gods, says—where, more than an analysis of the subject's feelings, certain demands of the object participate. So, we can think of the relations between object and subject not as a simple "confrontation", but rather as *a complex shared terrain where a dialectical dimension is established.* The intermediate space in such experience is highlighted, so that there cannot be an experience of the work or about the work, but only "with the work", and this "with" ("*mit*"), point of encounter, initiates what we can consider *the event* (Fragasso, 2001). The encounter with art is one of the "truth-events" (Badiou, 2000) that, as a rupture in the field of knowledge of the situation, is linked to the unsymbolized truth of the situation and that moves the life of a subject. In turn, within the field of aesthetics, it implies the idea of beauty, says Gadamer (1998), since it has the character of "event", of "happening" and being part of it. The idea of the beautiful, for Plato, implies "attraction of the beautiful" to itself, which demands and promotes participation (*metexis*); then, we can conclude that the aesthetic experience necessarily incorporates its participants. From these perspectives, the aesthetic experience is an event, it is an encounter: a *paradoxical place of encounter* where the subject *is* the object of art itself, as a *condition of mediation that enables this encounter*.

Freud's account in Athens shows that condition of possibility of aesthetic experience at the moment when the object ceases to be the Acropolis and becomes, as an "ambiguous object" (Oliveras, 2008), the object of that experience. I understand, then, that it is that *lost object*, between reality and fantasy, which is memory and nostalgia, and condition of strangeness: "There is an ominous effect, when the boundaries between fantasy and reality are blurred, when there appears before us as real something that we had taken for fantastic, when a symbol assumes the full operation and meaning of the symbolized" (Freud, 1919, p. 244), as the Acropolis may have been for Freud.

I propose to think of the aesthetic experience as a *border experience* between the forbidden and the permitted, as the last veil that art does not unveil. And it is precisely in that *hidden encounter* where the experience resides and the I of pleasure summoned takes us back to distant times in which reality is suspended and pleasure is dilated; the one who experiences it feels that he is held as if in a rocking arm. Memories are activated from the traces of "that unforgettable other of our prehistory" (Freud, 1896, p. 280), the other of the narcissistic reflex, the other that identifies me. It would be a temporary, "dialectical" regression outside pathology, to "times in which the ego had not yet clearly separated itself from the external world, nor from the Other" (Freud, 1919, p. 236). Times in which the self is not-self, ancient times where an unconscious reality is touched and, like an instantaneous vision, discovers a truth to consciousness, something of primordial times of the soul that have long since been overcome. Thus, the experience of estrangement is experience in a place of transition, where fantasies, desire, pleasure and play are admitted; a place where the beautiful and, in a certain way, the uncanny take place. A place where, especially, art takes place and where the experience itself is presented, which, even if only for an instant, transforms our existence.

0.5 Freud at the Acropolis according to some hypothetical premises

- If, on the Acropolis, Freud was part of an aesthetic experience and
- He does not accept to be part of it without doing so through reasoning.
- Then, we understand that Freud experienced a feeling of alienation by being part of that aesthetic experience in the Acropolis and not being able to resort to reason.

We understand that, from Freud's separation into *two persons,* which he himself describes as a split, a product of the denial of what he sees, this experience is triggered. And so, by means of associations, the signifying chain unfolds, from one memory to another, approaching remote zones that he seemed not to want to remember in a "repressive" effort—as he puts it—, and that he manages to associate through the disturbance of the memory. Freud thought that he did not believe in the existence of the Acropolis, but in reality, he was denying an ambitious desire: to get there someday, thus surpassing his father. A feeling of pity invaded him: to get there someday.

It is from his interpretation of the disturbance of memory and the admission of having experienced an alienation that the nucleus of truth emerges, also as an aesthetic experience.

We thus arrive at the central point of the aesthetic experience: alienating truth in which the self is not unique and coherent, a reality that deceives it, that by admitting the split, admits that I am also another (*car je est un autre,* in Rimbaud's words). The other becomes I and the I becomes alienated in the other, showing the ***dialectical function*** of alienation and separation and of the I/not-I from the times of identificatory jubilation, where the foundations of our aesthetic possibility reside, where we see ourselves, where we are looked at. Didi-Huberman (1997, p.13), goes even further by affirming that what we see "is not worth, does not live, in our eyes except for what looks at us [...] it is the split that separates in us what we see from what looks at us in an irremediable way. Therefore, it is necessary to start from the consideration that the act of seeing only unfolds by opening itself in two. We consider a modality of ***dialectical splitting*** that understands as structuring the admission of doubt, where the denial sustained in the non-pathological aspects of feelings of alienation would be throwing upon us the possibility of aesthetic experience. It is part of it a form of splitting of the ego and alienation, which give rise to experience, and to the irruption of the unconscious.

In estrangement something similar happens to certain "unusual phenomena" that make us doubt our perception. Freud analyzes them in the manner of mental mirages in which we want to recognize something as belonging to our ego or, in alienations, we want to exclude it. When this is clarified, we can see a fragment of something hidden that thus comes to light, threading fantasies and forgotten memories. Borges says: "What would I not give for memory (I had it and have lost it)", says Borges in "Elegy of an impossible memory" (Borges, 1976), memory and longing that we try to catch and search for in the enigma of life: "And we search for something else. We seek poetry; we seek life. And life is, I am sure, made of poetry. Poetry is not something strange: it is lurking, as we shall see, around the corner" (Borges, 2001).

Note

1 The underlining is the author's.

References

Agamben, G. (1995) *Homo sacer. Il potere sovrano e la nuda* vita, Turín, Einaudi.
Badiou, A. (2000) Presentación de la edición en castellano de El ser y el acontecimiento. Acontecimiento, 10(19–20), 11–25.
Borges, JL (2001) Arte poética, Barcelona, Editorial Crítica, pp. 15–35.
Borges, JL (1976) "Elegía de un recuerdo imposible" La moneda de hierro, Buenos Aires, Editorial Sudamericana.
Didi-Huberman, G (1997) Lo que vemos, lo que nos mira, Barcelona, Manantial.
Fragasso, L. (2001) Escritos y clases de estética y filosofía.
Freud, S. (1896) "Carta 52", Los orígenes del psicoanálisis, A. E., I.
Freud, S. (1914) El Moisés de Miguel Ángel, A. E., XIII.
Freud, S. (1919) "Lo ominoso", A. E., XVII.
Freud, S. (1927) "El porvenir de una ilusión", A. E., XXI.
Freud, S. (1936) "Carta a Romain Rolland" ('Una perturbación del recuerdo en la Acrópolis')", A. E., XXII.
Gadamer, H.G. (1998) La Actualidad De Lo Bello, S.A, Argentina, Paidós ibérica.
Goldstein, G. (2005) "La experiencia estética", Buenos Aires, del estante editorial.
Oliveras, E. (2008) "Theory of the Ambiguous Object", in Elena Oliveras (editor) Cuestiones de arte contemporáneo. Hacia un nuevo espectador en el siglo XXI, Buenos Aires, Emecé.

1 The Concept of Estrangement, Art and Aesthetics

1.1 Aesthetic experience and estrangement, an unsettling region (poetics of creativity)

Art has always been a subject of interest and has occupied, and still occupies, a preeminent place in life and in psychoanalysis. For Freud, the study of artistic productions from aesthetics, understood as "science of the beautiful" that designates the qualities of our feeling, is insufficient to account for the deep and enigmatic function of art and some experiences with art that produce violent or disconcerting emotions. Psychoanalysis, which deals with "other strata of the psychic life", to put it as Freud does in "The Uncanny", can account for some questions neglected by scholars of the "supreme effects" of art (Freud, 1919, p. 219). What characterizes these supreme effects produced by the encounter with art? What conditions of this encounter make the aesthetic experience possible?

The aesthetic experience, in terms of Alain Badiou (2000), is an encounter of the subject with the object of art with the character of an event, which implies, in my opinion, a form of non-pathological estrangement that includes creative processes. The estrangement is the core of the aesthetic experience; it is the affective state of non-pathological consequences and the condition of possibility of the experience. The encounter "between" subject and object, as an event, is the framework in which estrangement occurs. Such an event defines an "experience of the instant" which is the moment of surprise in the encounter with art or is an impact, lived as such, with direct repercussions on the body. It is a non-traumatogenic disruptive impact (Benyakar, 2006), in that it initiates a non-pathological estrangement. The estrangement, under these conditions as the core of the aesthetic experience, includes creative processes that deploy a "dimension of estrangement". In this "place" or dimension of estrangement, there are exchanges between subject and object, a dialectic, between reality and fantasy, between modes of psychic processes: between primary and secondary processes, between inside and outside, between what is one's own and what is strange, giving rise to creative processes related to tertiary processes. Thus, this state of estrangement configures a wide region of diffuse, but not indeterminate, borders. There opens the plot of what could

DOI: 10.4324/9781003591559-2

be called a topology of estrangement, where objects and subjects change their positions, unite in a "temporary fusion" that alienates them to the experience in a creative sense. That is, in the sense of the production of something unprecedented. And then they separate, they meet again reflexively. Under these conditions, something is produced in the poietic sense, in the sense of creating, of production. In estrangement there is a creative unreality, of production of something new. The subject of experience is open, in perceptual uncertainty, to the plurivocity of the object, which gives rise to metaphor. Something is something different from what it is, or from what it seems, and produces associations in the manner of free association, distant memories or descriptions and narratives that are poetic in character, insofar as they constitute an interpretation or construction whose framework is the encounter between the subject of experience and the object of art. Under these conditions aesthetic pleasure presents itself as a form of paradoxical pleasure, by admitting that something that seems astonishing can be like sustaining the beautiful and the disturbing, the Apollonian and the Dionysian, at the same time. This is part of the phenomenal field of aesthetic experience, and modes of pleasure that correspond to the state of estrangement. This paradoxical pleasure is a "way out" of estrangement, as an index of binding in a mode of psychic processing that accesses understanding as some formalization of the sensation and the state lived in the aesthetic experience.

1.1.1 *Freud's estrangement at the Acropolis*

As we have seen, in the "Letter to Romain Rolland ('A Disturbance of Memory at the Acropolis')" (Freud, 1936), Freud describes an "unusual" and enigmatic phenomenon that happens to him in Athens. In this situation there are questions that relate art, aesthetic experience and psychoanalysis, with the "feeling of alienation" or estrangement that Freud refers to and that precipitate questions that show that an aesthetic experience takes place there. An experience that could also be described as the sensation of "Aha, Erlebnis", that is, "Aha, I am here!" (Lacan, 1949). And I can't believe it. Freud's writing in Athens reveals that he cannot believe he is there, before the Acropolis of Athens, when he exclaims, "Then all this does indeed exist just as we learned it in school!" This forgetfulness or disbelief reveals the strange phenomenon that happens to him. The exemplary Freudian experience, referred to in the story, thus points out a starting point for the question that interrogates the aesthetic experience and estrangement.

Thus, Freud's experience on the Acropolis (1936, p. 209), as an aesthetic experience, has the character of an event and initiates a "sequence" as a "passage" to the "small experience" which appears as the feeling of estrangement described by Freud, which enables a space of experience that, in the conditions in which this passage takes place, assumes the institution of aesthetic experience. What happened to Freud, who contemplates as "situational apperception" a part of himself, externalized, as a component of the landscape, while another part of him does not admit reality and retains himself in doubt? The alienated experience at the Acropolis is analyzed by Freud in the field of the Oedipus. He determines that what produced his "little" experience was a pitying motion. The problem of the feeling of alienation, or estrangement, remains as a disturbing question, on which Freud decides to "forbid himself to elucidate further". Where Freud stops, he proposes to continue investigating, thinking about the strange and another reading of the feeling of estrangement as the core of the aesthetic experience.

What is called "a 'feeling of alienation' (*Entfremdungsgefühl*) or 'feeling of estrangement'", says Freud, are phenomena misunderstood (Freud, 1936, p. 218) outside of pathology, in the manner of "mental mirages". But investigating from other fields, we see that this estrangement appears as a condition of possibility of a modern aesthetic experience in which the objects of this experience move us and make us think; in Reimer's terms (in Steiner 2006, p. 25), *they* question us, they demand a reaction from us. Thus, in this state, the object, which in the beginning was the Acropolis, becomes an ambiguous, enigmatic object, which is the condition of art objects in the aesthetic experience: they are always something else, something else that goes beyond what they represent or present, given that their metaphorical potential opens the interpretation to the associations of those who are part of the experience. It is something of the "enigmatic" of art. This "state" implies the subject as part of the aesthetic experience itself. From this perspective of aesthetics, it is understood that the aesthetic experience implies the configuration of a "disturbing region", a place without men or gods, as Agamben (1995) says, and following Heidegger we highlight the hegemony of the intermediate space that implies an experience with the work "with" ("mit"), a meeting point, which we can consider the event. On his side, Gadamer argues that (Gadamer, 1998) that event implies the encounter with beauty since it has the character of "event", of "happening". However, the notion of event as an encounter with art provokes something more, since, as Badiou states in the "Presentation in English" of "Being and the Event", art is one of the four fields in which the advent of truth-events takes place. From this point of view, truth and art enter into relation, as an event, since for Badiou (2000) this implies a rupture in the field of knowledge of the situation that is linked to the non-symbolized truth of the situation itself. In these conditions, the encounter with art introduces something of that truth, which, as an aesthetic experience, is an event that makes a mark in the life of a subject and, in an unexpected way, potentially reorganizes his psychic economy.

Likewise, the experience of estrangement is an experience not only in a place of transition, where fantasies, desire, pleasure, and play circulate with their own legality, but also in the loosening of the ties of the ego with reality and the agencies, where the beautiful and the sinister occur. This state, estrangement, is a different mode of psychic functioning that is related to that of the dream, but in waking life, with the creative phantasy (of which

Freud speaks in "Writers and day-dreaming" 1908) and with the dimension of the game, which is pleasure and repetition of something beyond in the movement of the drive, which in certain conditions, promotes some rewriting or retracing, of something previously unmetabolized or symbolized. In this state, a fragment of truth emerges, as something real, which appears incarnated in the unexpected encounter with the object of art, resonance of the lost object, as a trace of *das ding*—"the thing"—and the sensorial perceptual complex of the other (as Freud refers to it in the "The Project for a scientific psychology" (1895). This is a very distinct sensation that has an effect on judgment, as it appears in the strange dimension of the screen memory, where the categories are "confused", as Freud says, since he affirms that it is a "sensation" that moves us in all those moments, and that "… undoubtedly it is a judgment and indeed a judgment of discernment, but these cases possess a very particular character, and the fact that what is sought is never remembered should not be neglected" (Freud, 1901, p. 257). It could be said that one does not find what was sought, but something other, something lost, something strange or alien to the world or to oneself.

Freud's account in Athens exposes the instant in which the event of the encounter with the object, the Acropolis, initiates the state of estrangement. In this condition of estrangement, the object ceases to be the Acropolis and becomes an ambiguous object that involves, beyond the beautiful, something of the ominous. Strangeness implies a state of unreality in relation to what is perceived, but outside of pathology; and this involves the beautiful and the ominous, the desired and the feared, by momentarily blurring the boundaries between fantasy and reality. In estrangement as the core of aesthetic experience, sensations promote a state in which one is awake, but it seems like a dream, a reverie, or a fantasy. Primary processes emerge in the midst of and alongside secondary processes and do not follow a single direction, as in the dream, but are "swinging" in an "in-between" that permeates the self of consciousness, accounting for a dialectical dimension, as a state of creativity. The psyche becomes "porous" and is affected by sensations. It opens up to the unfolding of tertiary processes that relate and limit the interplay of both the primary and the secondary (Green, 1995). This state, to which Gilbert J. Rose (1980) alludes, speaks of something like a reality with fluid edges between the self and the art object. Then, estrangement configures a zone, an intermediate space, whose permeable edges enable the aesthetic experience, a dimension in movement between the principle of reality and the principle of pleasure that could be called the "topology of estrangement". That "place" between the forbidden and the permitted, where the I of pleasure summoned up takes us back to distant times in a temporary, swinging, out of pathology, times where the I is not-I, where an unconscious reality is touched and reveals a truth to the conscience. I state in my aforementioned book that the aesthetic experience as the psychoanalytic experience implies the possibility of experiencing a truth (Goldstein, 2005).

1.1.2 *"The trace of a lost likeness"*

It is an "alienating" truth in which it becomes clear that the I is not unique and coherent, since its very consciousness is a reality that deceives it by admitting that the I is also another (*car je est un autre*, in Rimbaud's words). The other becomes self and the self becomes alienated in the other, showing the dialectical function of alienation and separation of self/non-self from the times of identification jubilation, where the foundations of our aesthetic possibility reside, where we see ourselves, where we are looked at. Didi-Huberman, scholar of aesthetics and contemporary art, quoting Joyce in what he called the: "ineluctable modality of the visible says that it is [...] like a going back to that antiquity that leads to the trace of a lost likeness." (1997, p. 13)

Such non-pathological modes of feelings of alienation open the subject to the possibility of aesthetic experience. In estrangement something similar happens to certain "unusual phenomena", such as *déjà vu, déjà raconté* or *fausse reconnaissance*, which make us doubt our perception. For Freud, it is a momentary admission of a fragment of truth, which, as in alienations, we wish to exclude. These alienations or estrangements, says Freud in his letter to Rolland, are "like 'sensations', but it is evident that they are complex processes, tied to certain contents and connected with decisions about the latter ..." (Freud, 1936, p. 218).

The subject is engaged in the experience in the face of something unexpected, either shock, or surprise. In those conditions in which estrangement is promoted, there are sensations that account for the subjective involvement and the emergence of the subject in this encounter. This instant is beyond words and differs from other experiences with art. In other words, it could be said that there is a discontinuity in the discourse. And that estrangement provokes a form of pleasure that accompanies the aesthetic experience and is its correlate; it is a complex, paradoxical pleasure. They are modes of pleasure that accompany the exteriorization of the estrangement that is being formalized with a charge of affection, in a feeling, in different tonalities, ominous, nostalgic, or erotic. Eros appears as a creative potential, in the sense of bonding, as a microscopic dimension in which some of these psychic states occur. Psyche and Eros are the parts of pleasure at play, involving the soul as mystical and psychic experience. In the meeting of these two terms, Eros and Psyche, Green sees an essential chapter of Freud's testament: "Eros is one of the members of a pair of forces and then states that Eros, life force, became a part of Psyche" (Green, 1997, p. 137), therefore "Eros, the force of the bond, "will bind at the same time the internal world—the psyche—and the relationship with the object situated in the external world, but formed by incorporation in the internal world" (Green, 1997, p. 137).

It can be said, then, that the aesthetic experience takes place from the encounter with the object of art of the order of the event, which triggers estrangement. The estrangement is the core of the aesthetic experience, its condition of possibility, whose temporal and physical correlate is the experience of the instant. This "instant" is a surprising, unexpected instant that produces an effect on the body directly as a jolt, or a sensation of immersion in a timeless time that detaches itself from chronological or dated time. The instant is experienced as a discontinuity that acquires a certain consistency. It is the expression of a privileged instant that separates itself from the chain of time. It is characterized by the loss of the notion of time, as Wagner's Parsifal expresses it in the enigmatic phrase "*Zum Raum wird hier die Zeit*" ("Here time becomes space"). In this state, experience unfolds its poetic dimension; this encounter with art touches the intimate fiber that moves the subject and makes the subject of experience emerge in an unknown dimension. Something of the unknowable emerges in a moment of truth.

In the aesthetic experience circulates an aesthetic pleasure, pleasure that we call paradoxical pleasure, because, following the ideas of André Green (Green, 1997), it promotes "chains that unfold according to a series of formations: the drive and its pulsion motions, the state of pleasure and its correlate, the displeasure and the desire expressed as a state of expectation and search, the fantasies, which organize the script of desire; "the erotic love language of sublimations" (Green, 1997, p. 251). Eros as a ligature is formalization, and the exit from a state of stupor by art, shock or amazement that leaves us beyond words. This complex interweaving of an aesthetic experience, as it is defined, is what makes this experience an encounter that moves the subject, and brings him closer to the Other, the strange, the alien, which can have a disturbing effect. For this reason, it is affirmed that what Freud defines as a feeling of estrangement is a transitory state, which promotes, in these conditions, an openness to experience those accounts for the singularity of each subject. The encounter of the subject of experience with art in estrangement as an aesthetic experience produces complex, intersubjective, intrapsychic exchanges with the object, which, due to their characteristics, make the emergence of the subject as a lost object and of the unconscious as a poetic condition.

This encounter with the object determines an effect on the subject in the context of the aesthetic experience, it involves a crossing of something, in the manner of a resistance, (which may or may not be achieved) and has the character of an encounter with something unexpected, or thought of as impossible. Something of "the lost" in Freud and of "the real" in Lacan come into play. The conditions explored so far describe phenomena and characteristics of the subject's experience with the object of experience that involve the feeling of estrangement (Freud, 1923), the relation of the *unknown* according to Rosolato (1978), and *alienation* (Lacan, 2006). This estrangement, as it marks the crossing of an aesthetic experience, implies the possibility of mobilizing defenses and promoting the deployment of creative processes—as poetic disruption—and thus mobilizes unconscious motions, providing clues for new inscriptions in the experiential plot.

1.2 The aesthetic experience: From the philosophers of Greek Antiquity to the twentieth century

We review here some concepts on aesthetics and aesthetic experience from philosophy, which support the central thesis of the book in relation to knowledge and, in a particular way, the dialectic between sensation and reason as a paradoxical dimension, which sustains the conceptualization of a "sensitive thought". It also contributes to the notion of what happens in the phenomenon of estrangement, as associations or imagination. The antecedents of the relation between art, aesthetics, philosophy, and the knowledge of the world can be traced back to Plato and Aristotle, who postulated different theses. While Plato had tenaciously fought against the consecration of the poet as the master of truth and of art as a vehicle of knowledge, Aristotle allowed himself to value mimetic art not only on the basis of some specific function but also in view of a peculiarly aesthetic effect: the generation of a certain type of pleasure. The main reflections on art appear, in Aristotle, with the notes of presumably incomplete classes known as *Poetics*.[1] These meant the consolidation, in the Greek world, of a new tradition based on writing, which was superimposed on the oral poetic-mimetic culture. This gives poetry a place of privilege over history and even, in a certain sense, on a par with philosophy. In a way this represents the overcoming of the ancient Greek oral culture, the Homeric.

It was Aristotle who coined the term Katharsis, in relation to tragic poetry in particular, and thus, insofar as it is associated with the ultimate goal of tragic drama, it has been understood as a reference to a certain process of purging or purification of emotions, which would provoke a certain degree of relief and consequent pleasure. The study of this perspective gave rise to two new interpretative currents: one links Katharsis to a certain type of intellectual clarification, and the other tries to account for the pleasure that tragedy arouses. Without going into details about them, it is clear that the ways of interpreting Aristotelian statements refer the discharge to a particular mode of access to knowledge of the world and/or to a particular form of access to pleasure. Moreover, it can be inferred that, already from these first glances, the human being has always tried to understand and communicate the "purely aesthetic element" and its particular qualities. In this regard, Lear says, quoting Aristotle

> That very thing, by the way, is perforce experienced not only by those inclined to piety but also by those subject to terror and, in general, by those possessed by passion, and the rest, insofar as such emotions may affect each one, and perforce in all there will be some purification [katharsis] and relief mingled with pleasure.
>
> (Aristotle, 2009: 1342a 10–15, p. 470)"

Lear, (1988) in attempting to describe the type of pleasure associated with *katharsis*, argues:

> ...the poet, according to Aristotle, plays the same role with regard to emotions that the skeptic plays with regard to knowledge. In this sense, the tragic drama opens the eyes of the spectator to certain emotional possibilities that are not considered in real life
>
> (p. 324).

It is interesting to note the cut on Aristotelian notions, which refer not only to a particular experience of pleasure, but also to a specific relationship with reality, where the experience—of tragedy in this case—, thanks to the imagination and the distance from "real life", allows the "happening of extreme emotional events", which enjoy a certain disbelief by the spectator, which locate other characteristics attributed to the aesthetic experience in this book, such as "paradoxical" pleasure and the feeling of estrangement or distancing from reality. Aristotle originally argues that the poet must produce, at the same time, "compassion and awe" (Aristotle, 1990, p. 63).

Already in Modernity, preponderant value is given to subjectivity and there are several referents within philosophy that refer to the intersubjective value of art. Modern man is interested in the sensory world and a movement toward the secularization of thought begins to take shape. Faith in God, which had guaranteed true knowledge during the Middle Ages, weakens as science advances. The rise of Cartesian doubt is an example of how definitive truths begin to crumble. From this it is understandable that the concept of *objective beauty* that had prevailed for so many centuries begins to decay. The appearance of aesthetics as a specific discipline through A. T. Baumgarten in the middle of the eighteenth century, refers to knowledge created from the sensitivity of man and a new valuation of the singular. With the influence of Baumgarten and Edmund Burke, Immanuel Kant is led to a systematization of aesthetics for the modern world. The appearance of *Critique of Judgment* (Kant, 2005/1790) inaugurates what could be called modern aesthetics.

Kant opens the way to the discipline of aesthetics, through a critique. He sustains the conditions by means of which it justifies itself by giving an account of its *a priori* or of the operations of thought and judgment that make it possible. Herein lies the originality of Kantian thought, as his three critiques attest. Kant makes a transcendental critique. This differs from a world system in that it does not establish the answers regarding knowledge, morality or beauty. Likewise, it does not answer the question as to why a given work provokes the emergence of certain feelings -since its territory is not empirical but transcendental. It concentrates on the establishment of the operations of reason or of the subject that make possible any knowledge, moral act or aesthetic experience.

Kant was the first modern philosopher to make his aesthetic theory a fundamental part of the philosophical system. He postulated that an object that no longer has finality or function, but due to a certain totality seems to have been made to be understood, has finality in its form and thus evokes aesthetic satisfaction (Rose, 1980). This formal finality leads to a "free play of the imagination", a pleasure that depends on the harmony between imagination and understanding. Kant saw in form a modality of perception and cognition that modeling sensations, turning them into a subjective and systematic experience of reality, especially in relation to the spatio-temporal order.

Kant establishes a difference between "judgments of sensation", "practical judgments", and "aesthetic judgments" to substantiate his propositions on aesthetic experience. The pleasure obtained from the object does not depend on its properties nor on that for which that object is a means, i.e., its practical character, all these things remain outside the aesthetic experience. If we were to pay attention to what the thing is, we would be producing a judgment of knowledge. In the aesthetic judgment, on the other hand, we turn our attention to the feeling of pleasure we derive from it. But this is not related to the sensation of the object—for we would thus be in the field of a judgment of sensation—nor to the concept of the good since this would lead us to that of the moral. This remains outside the aesthetic experience. Thus said, and remembering that Kant defines as *experience* any meaningful relation between the subject and the object, it can be understood that the subject lives an experience when "the object affects him in a particular way and enriches the meanings of his world" (Capdevila i Castells, 2005, p. 140).

The paradox is that the process of aesthetic judgment seems to begin in a given object—without ultimately concerning it—and end in the feeling of the subject, but is autonomous of this particular mode of feeling or of the particular inclinations of the subject. Indeed, the pleasure of aesthetic judgment, "originates in some way in the particular relation between representation and feeling" (p. 140). From this statement it follows that "aesthetic pleasure does not originate in the immediate perception of an object, but consists in the result of another experience: aesthetic pleasure is the experience of another experience" (Capdevila i Castells, 2005, p. 140). The specificity of Kant's research lies in a fundamental discovery that allows the foundation of an autonomous dimension where aesthetic experience takes place.

A development that leads to another consideration of reason in relation to art is the one addressed by Hegel. Aesthetics is constituted, for Hegel, in a moment of expression and self-knowledge of the Spirit in its sensible form, being part of the process of self-reflection of modernity. At the same time, it resonates in the notion that we propose of "**sensitive thought**" since, "art is the sensible (sensitive) appearance of the idea", says Hegel; but at the same time the work of art does not belong to the order of immediate sensibility.

Walter Biemel affirms that *Kant wanted to demonstrate this change by insisting on "the special capacity of the work of art to arouse a disinterested interest". The work of art claims our attention not as something that corresponds to our desires, but as something that puts in concordance, imagination and intelligence. He says that Hegel "explains this change operated in the domain of sensitivity, showing that the work of art needs sensitivity. In order to be realized, the work of art makes use of sensibility, but at the same time it elevates us above it. Rather, the work of art teaches us that what we believed to be reality can be overcome"*.

In this quote, the author establishes two clear references to aspects of the aesthetic experience and the work of art that are taken up again in this book. The need for an encounter with the object on a sensitive plane but which requires a movement of the subject, to "go beyond complacency, desire", and create a new reality from the imagination, as Biemel explains. Adds Biemel (1962) quoting Hegel that: "Comparing it with the approximation of immediate sensible existence … the appearance of art has the advantage that it is an appearance that surpasses itself and indicates something spiritual that must appear through it" (p. 14). Thus, Hegel puts the sensible world in relation to thought and, in this sense, the effect of giving meaning to sensible experience, which sets in motion the activity of thought. This reflection is related to what I propose in this book from the aesthetic experience, by promoting an opening, which unfolds potentially creative processes, in a sense of new, mutative and resignifying inscriptions of what has already been lived.

Kantian aesthetics had a great impact on the philosophers who succeeded him. Among many in this path, and of particular interest, is Schopenhauer (1818), since one of the most suggestive features of Schopenhauerian aesthetics is consideration of art as the most adequate means for the knowledge of the world: The content or object of art [Schopenhauer notes in his Lessons …] … "is that which remains alien to, and independent of, all relations; that which is properly essential to the world; that which is truly essential to the world; that which is independent of all relations … "is that which remains alien to, and is independent of all relations; that which is properly essential to the world; the true content of all phenomena; that which is not subject to change and is known once and for all with a single truth; in a word: the ideas, which are the immediate and adequate objectification of *the thing in itself*." (emphasis in original)

Just as, according to Schopenhauer, the "concept" arises from a process of abstraction whose raw material is constituted by the multiple intuitive representations acquired by an individual, in the case of art, the matter is quite different. Toward the end of Book II of MVR, in §27 of *The World as Will and Representation*, and after affirming that understanding is at the service of the will, Schopenhauer points out a caveat: it is the case that "in some particular men knowledge is capable of subtracting itself from that servitude, throwing off its yoke and, free from all the ends of willing, subsisting by itself as a clear mirror of the world: hence art is born …".

Knowledge through art is thus contrasted with both everyday knowledge and scientific knowledge.

Later in the century, reflection on the subject, reason, and aesthetics will lead to other kinds of theoretical explorations. From the development of Kant and the direction it finds in Schelling, aesthetics and art will acquire a progressive "relative autonomy" being part of the spheres of philosophical reason. With Hegel, on the other hand, the science of art is a constitutive moment of reason in the West. At the end of the century, aesthetic reflection embraces human existence itself and the way in which individuality and its problems and paradoxes are affirmed, of which psychoanalysis is an example. We can think, following these authors, and regarding that experience, that the subject will find both the risk of his negation in the relation with the social world (alienation), and the discovery of the shadow, with Nietzsche, which is part of himself and with which he is in permanent conflict. In each of these authors, their works represent a key that leaves open the possibility of conquering and producing another socio-political (Marx) or subjective world through creation and experience (Nietzsche).

It is interesting to recover with Schelling what is observed in a radical attempt to articulate reason split from sensuality. Art as artifice is criticized in order to give rise, finally, to an intrinsic relation between natural and artistic beauty. This is achieved—according to Schelling—through a true aestheticization of philosophy. In this way:

> … art is constituted as the first place in which the intimate, intrinsic unity of the Self and Nature, of the Subject and the Object, of the Conscious and the Unconscious is manifested. And it is this unity, laboriously acquired through the philosophical gaze, that manifests itself immediately, **prediscursively**, on the aesthetic plane. Within this conceptual apparatus, the aesthetic genius presents itself … as the place of passage between the unconscious and the conscious.
>
> (Vercellone, 2004, p. 17).

This activity of mediation and suture is carried out by the "genius" called to translate the unconscious into the conscious, the work being its main resource of subjectivation as well as its contact with the absolute, which establishes its condition of possibility. Given this condition (the relationship between genius and the absolute), the mediation between nature and culture will be affected through the work of art, constituting a direct expression of the absolute as such and its unconscious dimension. Schelling's and, more specifically, Nietzsche's developments directly allude, in the philosophical field, to the capacity of aesthetics, and especially of aesthetic experience, to knot paradoxical aspects of human experience that will be taken up again in Freudian developments on art from a psychoanalytical perspective.

1.3 The unknown, estrangement and the condition of knowledge

1.3.1 Russian Formalism: Estrangement and poetic language

Formalism was born in pre-revolutionary Russia at the beginning of the 20th century as an avant-garde linguistic-literary current that opposed the understanding of language as a simple means of communication and literature as a merely representative art. Its most representative referent was Viktor Shklovski (also Chklovski) and his work, "Art as artifice" (coined by Chklovski in 1925; *Искусссmво как прием*). He contributes the concept of deviation or *estrangement* (остранение). He argued that everydayness made us "lose the freshness of our perception of objects", that is, it made everyday life automated and postulates art as salvation from automation. His technique consists in making objects strange, in "creating complicated forms, increasing the difficulty and extension of perception, since, in aesthetics, the process of perception is an end in itself and, therefore, must be prolonged". This trend was later persecuted by Stalinism and disappeared from Eastern Europe in 1930.

There are links between Russian formalism and its postulation about estrangement and psychoanalysis, through Lacan's references to Jakobson, who belonged to this movement and developed his theories in the United States until 1939. As a literary movement with implications for linguistics, it can be said that its developments are divided into two stages, but for the purposes of this synthesis of the background of our notion, those contained in the first stage are relevant.

According to Eidelberg (2010), certain postulates of this movement are the foundation of some of the Lacanian definitions of language and analytical interpretation. Since language is an artifice, according to its founders, literary language must be poetic—whether written in prose or poetry—and as distinct from everyday language. Hence, according to Eidelberg, the sense that Lacan (quote) imposes on his definition of **analytic intervention as poetic**: that its utterances do not correspond to expected everyday language. Thus, estrangement has the correspondence of surprising or deviating from the automatic use of language in everyday life and promotes a "fresh" approach to objects.

On the other hand, the authors' reference to language as relevant in terms of understanding how it is made and how it works (its use), of addressing how the word plays in it at the different levels immanent to the text—and not paying attention to "what it means" in everyday terms—, also refers to the postulates about the formalization of language. It is evident that, in this theory, the sense of estrangement is again salvaged as the action of estrangement, as the intention of forcing the reader to decenter himself from the norm, from the everyday, and from there to reflect, to question that which fits into the customary definitions of reality. As in anthropology, formalist estrangement is a tool for accessing the subject's active perception of the world around him.

Pedro Serra (2015) advances in the study of the notion of estrangement from aesthetic theories. He locates the notion of estrangement as a "psychoanalytic theoretical object" in its definition through the Freudian ***unheimlich*** and raises the possibility of thinking about it in relation to the notion of "art as artifice" (coined by Shklovski in 1925).

Serra says:

> The imagination that Chklovski seeks to objectify by means of a concept has, at once, a name. Here is the place where his analytic produces a synthesis of the two modes of imagination: there are two types of images: the image as a practical means of thinking, as a means of grouping objects; and the poetic image, a means of reinforcing the impression. The name of this other faculty, as we see, is that of poetic imagination. All this is well known. But what I would like to emphasize is the syntagm "means of reinforcement of the impression", a syntagm that describes no longer an experiential mode of attribution of meaning -that would be the case of practical imagination-, but a mode of sensory experience.
>
> (Serra, 2015, p. 33).

Serra highlights the dichotomy between sensitive perception and automatism, typical of the proposal of Russian aesthetic formalism, and thus establishes an opposition between everyday life and art. Just as in mundane life a sensation is repeated until anesthesia, in art, the artist "*presents an object as if he were seeing it for the first time or presents an event as if it were happening for the first time*," says Shklovski (1978). According to Serra, the aesthetic experience lies in this fiction—"*comme si*", "*as if*"—of a first vision and occurrence (outside of pathology). In other words, the properly aesthetic moment of art is the repetition of a singularity. "Here is the 'difficulty', as he sees it, of art, of the poetic imagination: the fiction of the 'sensation' is the production of a 'sensation' more intense than the 'sensation' lived", (Serra, 2015, p. 33). And for this to be so, art has to put its cognitive dimension in suspension.

Thus, the crux of art is vision and not recognition; it is the production of sensations and not of meaning. Its purpose is poetic imagination, as the creation of a particular perception of the object, not its recognition or the compression of a meaning.

On the other hand, Serra, in his article, resorts to the notions of "Epiphany and Late Style" to complement what he defines as conditions of aesthetic experience. With Epiphany he refers to the idea of "apparition" or "manifestation" referring to an experiential mode in which something becomes present abruptly, a sudden manifestation of presence. Here he differs from the formalist model in that he opposes the "synchronization" between form and space. Since he argues that this synchronization is akin to automatism, the *epiphany* being necessary and complementary to the necessary estrangement in the aesthetic experience. Thus, he alludes to moments of epiphany, moments of intensity, where art *becomes present*.

Finally, he alludes to a modification of the perception of time in the aesthetic experience. He states: As Shklovski says, "The object is not perceived as a part of space, but so to speak, in its continuity. Poetic language satisfies these conditions .... In other words, the 'appearance' of the object presupposes, in addition, the 'absence' of space. It is a paradoxical experience. The materials that make up the 'substance of expression' are those that allow the manifestation of content in space" (Serra, 2015, p. 35).

This particular perception of time in the encounter with the art object, within the framework of an aesthetic experience, is broadly compatible with the notion of event, as Badiou asserts, also quoted by Moty Benyakar.

The alteration of the perception of time, linked to the notion of intensity and event, supposes "a sort of 'altered consciousness'" that "agonizes absence and presence", as Adorno states, quoted by Serra (2005, p. 35). It thus alludes to a modality of "the strange" where a sort of "separation" is assumed, referring to being in, but separated from the present.

1.3.2 *On estrangement as a condition of knowledge*

The question about art in general and about the aesthetic experience in particular has always been within the field of philosophy, but it has also been the focus of the concern of artists, anthropologists, sociologists, and psychologists. One of them is the American pragmatist, John Dewey.

In his work "Art as Experience", Dewey (1934/2008) concludes that in order to interpret his thought on art, it is necessary to refer to a superior philosophical—and epistemological—category called Experience, which will be in consonance with aesthetics: a quality that—according to Dewey—gives shape and consistency to the concept of aesthetic experience. Experience as man's experience is a determining factor in the meaning of art for Dewey.

Dewey approaches the concept of art by referring to the individual aspects of the human being, in order to, once these have been elucidated, be able to approach the concept of aesthetic experience. He speaks first of feeling, as a step after simple perception. The second aspect is knowledge, about which he clarifies that it is actually a pseudo-knowledge, since it consists, at least at the beginning, in a basic handling of information.

Man, whom Dewey baptizes as "the living creature", begins his encounter with the work of art from a feeling about some degree of beauty. In this process, man must come into contact with his environment and undergo a series of "transformations"—actions, hence the author's pragmatism. This alludes to the transformation of the artist's inner thoughts and feelings through the modification of an external and objective material, establishing new relationships and evoking new emotional responses. Finally, the work of art is the result or, in the author's terms, "the consummation" of an aesthetic experience. Such an experience culminates or is consummated when the individual finds meaning in the situation experienced, whether induced or accidental. At that moment, at the end or consummation of an experience, another one begins immediately, thus weaving continuous chains of minuscule experiences" (Dewey, 1934/2008, p. 99).

In philosophical terms, it could be asserted that estrangement, as a "prosaic experience of rupture with the given", is a condition of philosophizing. From estrangement, questions arise and, from there, concepts are created. In this way, estrangement is linked to the possibility of knowing.

Imre Lakatos called *methodological estrangement* as the "specific experience of generating a type of knowledge about the human being and any of its productions, which in turn conceives such products as components that constitute the producer", as Eduardo Álvarez Pedrosian recalls in his article "The experience of estrangement" (2009). In these terms, in addition to the specificity of the Lakatosian concept, it is worth paying attention to the fact that this concept has an intersubjectivist foundation: it is knowledge generated by the subject, from the position of being part of the field of knowledge. It is one of the most widespread strategies in the field of human sciences and it aims to access singular phenomena. It is a strategy of knowledge construction that seeks to build an objectification from the particular.

Álvarez Pedrosian says: "It is always about the same thing, the astonishment that triggers a cognitive process and the way of taking charge or not of this process" (2009, p. 65). In the case of methodological estrangement, it is the chronicler, the theorist (*theorós*) who observes, relates, and then reflects, constructing knowledge. In this posture, astonishment and estrangement are conditions for new knowledge. Thus, in philosophical terms, estrangement, as astonishment, is the trigger of a process of transformation, of a singular or subjective "intellectual adventure". Now, while the previous paragraphs allude to the link of estrangement with *logos*—as knowledge—the experience of estrangement is, Platonically, intimately linked to *pathos*, understood as a mute admiration (Wittgenstein), something that cannot be put into words. The social sciences and psychology in particular have tried, in recent decades, to address this dimension of feeling, outside the cognitive plane, which constitutes the experience of estrangement. Along the way, several possible scenarios have been constructed to establish answers, psychoanalysis being one of them.

On the other hand, estrangement as a method of access to knowledge is at the core of anthropology as a research strategy. Estrangement, in order to know different cultural or social practices, is a condition of its disciplinary constitution. As Álvarez Pedrosian states: "The pair identity/alterity, the question of the Other, the way of understanding and explaining a way of life, has been throughout the different theoretical matrices the channel of transmission of the gaze provoked by the experience of estrangement" (p. 65).

Thus, it becomes evident that estrangement as a state allows the opening to new processes of knowledge, sensibility, and perception that enable access to otherness. It is a weighted and systematized tool to build new subjective knowledge and, from there, new regularities that support theories.

1.3.3 *Art and reflection: The aesthetics of reception in Jauss*

Another of the central thinkers on aesthetic experience, Hans Jauss, brings together in his theory of aesthetics, the search for knowledge and enjoyment as a mode of access to the world, as a mode of reflection, untied from the question of aesthetic pleasure.

In 17th-century religious poetry, he explains, jouissance alluded to "participating in God" in an act in which the believer was immediately assured of his presence. In Goethe's *Faust*, Jauss continues, finally the concept of jouissance could be extended to all levels of experience, up to the highest longing for knowledge (from the vital jouissance of the person, through the jouissance of action and conscious jouissance, to the jouissance of creation). "Of these high flights of meaning nothing is recognized anymore", Jauss points out (2002, p. 35). Once, jouissance as a mode of appropriation of the world and of self-consciousness legitimized dealings with art, just as today aesthetic experience is considered genuine only if it leaves behind all pleasure and rises to the realm of aesthetic reflection.

Jauss differs from Theodor Adorno, who claims that those who seek and find pleasure in works of art are banal or bourgeois. On the other hand, in Jauss's arguments, we find, for example, criticism of the Marxist theory of literature, for having reduced aesthetic pleasure "to being a reflection, and therefore, to the mimetic ideal of bourgeois realism. He then expects from the passive subject a recognition of objective reality (...) but always with the aim of educating the subject against his inclination to aesthetic pleasure and transforming his empathy and identification into a reflexive and critical attitude" (Jauss, 2002, p. 37).

Jauss' position, as a faithful exponent of reception aesthetics, has so far dealt with the problem referring to consumer literature with respect to the so-called masterpieces, from a primary negativity toward a more pleasurable familiarity, but arguing that this approach presupposes that "*aesthetic reflection is the foundation of all reception and thus participates in the surprisingly unanimous ethics that has been imposed on art theory vis-à-vis primary aesthetic experience*" (Jauss, 2002, p. 37). In this line of argument, Jauss, then wonders where primary aesthetic experience lies and how aesthetic enjoyment is distinguished from sense pleasure. Artistic experience was by no means consolidated by opposition to knowing and acting. "The cognitive virtuality of aesthetic enjoyment, which still plays a role in Goethe's Faust as opposed to abstract conceptual knowledge, was only abandoned in the nineteenth century with the transition to the autonomy of art" (Jauss, 2002, p. 39).

According to Jauss' position, in aesthetic experience, jouissance is distinguished from simple sense pleasure—as almost all aesthetic theories since the Kantian doctrine of disinterested satisfaction confirm—by the *distance between the self and the object, or aesthetic distance*. Unlike the theoretical attitude, which likewise presupposes distancing, in the act of aesthetic enjoyment the contemplator frees himself from his ties to everyday praxis by means of the imaginary. In the primary process of aesthetic experience, the imaginary is not yet an object, but, as Sartre showed, an act of distancing and formalization of the representative consciousness. *The imaginative consciousness has to deny the factual world of objects in order to be able to create for itself, by means of the aesthetic sign, a configuration of words, images, or sounds.*

In this vision, which registers the state of pleasure of the aesthetic experience that will be developed in this book, the attitude of aesthetic enjoyment frees man from his daily chores and enables him for "another experience (…) Liberation through aesthetic experience can take place on three levels: for the productive consciousness, by engendering the world as its own work; for the receptive consciousness, by taking advantage of the possibility of perceiving the world in another way (…)" (Jauss, 2002, p. 41). But, above all, and finally, by showing how the subjectivity of the observer opens up to intersubjective experience. The aesthetic experience, as a state of pleasure, is therefore always a liberation as evidenced in the Aristotelian doctrine of *catharsis*. The consideration for the imaginary frees the spectator from practical interests to activate the pure affections, says Jauss.

Finally, Jauss proposes three fundamental concepts of the aesthetic tradition: *poiesis*, *aisthesis*, and *catharsis* to refer to the aesthetic experience. *Poiesis*, understood as a *poetic capacity*, designates the fundamental aesthetic experience that man, through the production of art, can satisfy his universal need to find himself at home in the world, depriving the outside world of its elusive strangeness, making the work his own, and obtaining in this activity a knowledge that is distinguished from both the conceptual knowledge of science and the instrumental praxis of the mechanical craft. *Aisthesis* denotes a change, where we find the fundamental aesthetic experience that a work of art can renew the perception of things, and where intuitive knowledge is opposed to the primacy of conceptual knowledge. Finally, *catharsis* designates the aesthetic experience that the beholder, in the reception of art, can be liberated from a partiality of practical life interests through aesthetic satisfaction, and be led toward a communicative or action-oriented identification. These aspects are linked to the Kantian definition of aesthetic pleasure as "experience of an experience", insofar as it is a way of finding a new, enriching sense of one's own world. In this book, this aspect is central, as the development of new senses, of new representations, unpublished, will be exposed as part of the intrinsic potential of the aesthetic experience.

Note

1 Aristotle, (2009) *Poetics*, Buenos Aires, Ediciones Colihue, Colecc. Colihue Clásica (Translation from Ancient Greek by Eduardo Sinnott).

References

Agamben, G. (1995) Homo sacer. Il potere sovrano e la nuda vita, Turín, Einaudi.
Álvarez Pedrosian, E. (2009) "The experience of estrangement". Paper presented at the VIII Reunión de Antropología del Mercosur (RAM): Diversidad y Poder en América Latina, Buenos Aires, September 29–October 2, 2009.
Aristotle, (2009) *Poetics*, Buenos Aires, Ediciones Colihue, Colecc. Colihue Clásica (Translation from Ancient Greek by Eduardo Sinnott).
Aristotle, (1990) Rhetoric, Madrid, Gredos. Translation by Quintín Racionero.
Badiou, A. (2000) Presentación de la edición en castellano de El ser y el acontecimiento. Acontecimiento, 10(19–20), 11–25.
Benyakar, M. (2006) Lo Disruptivo. Amenazas individuales y colectivas. El psiquismo ante guerras, terrorismo y catástrofes sociales, Buenos Aires, Ed. Biblos.
Biemel, W. (1962) "Hegel's Aesthetics", *Convivium, pp. 13–14.*
Capdevila i Castells, P (2005) Experiencia estética y hermenéutica. Tesis Doctoral, Universidad de Barcelona.
Didi-Huberman, G. (1997) Lo que vemos, lo que nos mira, Barcelona, Manantial.
Dewey, J (1934/2008) El arte como experiencia. Barcelona: Ed Paidós Ibérica
Eidelberg, A. (2010) Extrañamiento Formalista e Interpretación Psicoanalítica: http://www.aacademica.org/000-031/736
Freud, S. (1895) A Project for a Scientific Psychology (Standard Edition, Vol. 1, pp. 283–397), London, Hogarth.
Freud, S. (1901) The Psychopathology of Everyday Life: Forgetting, Slips of the Tongue, Bungled Actions, Superstitions and Errors. (The Standard Edition of the Complete Psychological Works of Sigmund Freud 6:vii-296), London.
Freud, S. (1919) "The 'Uncanny'". The Standard Edition of the Complete Psychological Works of Sigmund Freud, London, Hogarth Press and the Institute of Psycho-Analysis, pp. 217–256.
Freud, S. (1923) "El yo y el ello". Tomo XIX, O.C. Amorrortu.
Freud, S. (1936) "Carta a Romain Rolland" ('Una perturbación del recuerdo en la Acrópolis')", Tomo XXII, O.C. Amorrortu.
Gadamer, H. G. (1998) La Actualidad De Lo Bello, Argentina, Paidós ibérica.
Goldstein, G. (2005) La experiencia estética, Buenos Aires, del estante editorial.
Green, A. (1995) La metapsicologia revisitada, Buenos Aires, Editorial Eudeba
Green, A. (1997) Las Cadenas de Eros: Actualidad de lo Sexual, Buenos Aires, Amorrortu.
Jauss, H. R. (2002) Pequeña apología de la experiencia estética, Buenos Aires, Paidós, p. 35.
Kant, I. (2005/1790) Crítica del Juicio, Buenos Aires, Losada.
Lacan, J. (1949) Communication Zurich: "The mirror stage as the formator of the self (je) as it reveals itself to us in the psychoanalytic experience".
Lacan, J. (2006) "El sujeto y el otro: la alienación", in El seminario de Jacques Lacan. Libro 11, Los cuatro conceptos fundamentales del psicoanálisis, cap. XVI, Buenos Aires, Paidós.
Lear, J. (1988) "Katharsis". Phronesis, 33(3), 297–326.
Rose, G.J. (1980) The Power of Form, Nueva York, International Universities Press.
Rosolato, G. (1978) La relación de desconocido, Madrid, Ediciones Petrel.
Schopenhauer, A. (2005) The World as Will and Idea, trans. López de Santa María), Madrid, Trotta, p. 207.
Serra, P. (2005) "Strangeness, epiphany and late style". *El hilo de la fábula*. Annual review of the Center for Comparative Studies (15), p. 33.
Steiner, G. (2006) La idea de Europa, La cultura como invitación, Fondo de cultura económica, mexico d. f. p 25
Vercellone, F. (2004) Aesthetics of the 19th Century, Madrid, Ed. Machado, p. 17.

2 The Aesthetic Experience at the Beginning of the Psyche

2.1 Psychoanalysis and aesthetics

2.1.1 Aesthetics and estrangement in psychoanalytic theory

The term "aesthetics" has been changing its meaning through the different periods, theories, and authors who have approached this field. Not surprisingly, from the very moment the term is coined by Baumgarten in his work *Philosophical Reflections on Poetry* (1735), it refers to a kind of "confused knowledge" of the sensitive material which is opposed to the clear and distinct knowledge of the time, leaving a dimension open to different interpretations about the relationship between knowledge and sensations that are put in contact or opposed depending on the author who theorizes on aesthetics or aesthetic experience.

In this line, Rancière (2013) states that psychoanalysis is sustained by what he calls an "aesthetic unconscious" that arises from an "aesthetic regime". This regime, which is not temporally specific (beginning with *Oedipus Rex* and reappearing periodically until it becomes dominant in the "aesthetic revolution" in modernity), is a form of thought that can be identified by its constitutive "identity of opposites", which he considers an extension of the opposition between "pathos" and "logos", between sensation and reason; between the primary process and the need to grant it rationality and coherence through the operations of the secondary process. Thus, the "aesthetic revolution" or "aesthetic regime" to which he alludes is a revolution in which "an ordered set of relations between the visible and the invisible, knowledge and action, activity and passivity" are abolished.

I will now develop the relevant psychoanalytic concepts to explicit the theoretical foundations of estrangement as a condition of possibility of aesthetic experience, where this tension between opposites becomes a recurrent pattern and constitutes a basis for the understanding of "aesthetic experience" and creativity as a paradoxical concept within psychoanalytic theory.

The connection between the unconscious and artistic creation was present in Freudian texts from the very beginning of his work; this explains

DOI: 10.4324/9781003591559-3

why artists were the first to value the new contributions and discoveries of psychoanalysis: in 1895, one of the only voices in Vienna to publicly recognize the importance of the "Studies on Hysteria" as the prelude to a new psychology was that of Alfred von Berger, poet, literary critic, and director of the Imperial Theater in Vienna (Kris, 1946). In contrast, the reception by Viennese medicine and official science was negative, an understandable reaction considering the positivist tradition of the time. In "Creative writers and day-dreaming" of 1908, Freud considers art—like dreams, daydreams, and children's games—as a product of the artist's unconscious fantasy, whose purpose is to gratify repressed and unsatisfied desires:

> ... every child at play behaves like a creative writer, in that he creates a world of his own, or, rather, re-arranges the things of his world in a new way which pleases him
>
> (p. 143)

> ... As people grow up, then, they cease to play, and they seem to give up the yield of pleasure which they gained from playing. But whoever understands the human mind knows that hardly anything is harder for a man than to give up a pleasure which he has once experienced. Actually, we can never give anything up; we only exchange one thing for another ... instead of playing, he now phantasies
>
> (p. 145)

> ... The motive forces of phantasies are unsatisfied wishes, and every single phantasy is the fulfilment of a wish, a correction of unsatisfying reality
>
> (p. 146)

> ... And now for the creative writer. You will remember how I have said [p. 145 f.] that the day-dreamer carefully conceals his phantasies from other people because he feels he has reasons for being ashamed of them... when a creative writer presents his plays to us or tells us what we are inclined to take to be his personal day-dreams, we experience a great pleasure, and .... his innermost secret; the essential ars poetica ...
>
> (p. 153)

This relationship between psychoanalysis and aesthetics outlined in Freudian writing was taken up again by Rancière in his text, "The aesthetic unconscious" (2009). The author refers to several previous essays that address this interaction: in particular Otto Rank on dreams and poetry, and the works of Herbert Marcuse and the Frankfurt School, and focuses his thoughts on the question of the role that aesthetics has played in the constitution of Freudian thought.

Rancière will repeat this gesture by defining aesthetics not as a discipline endowed with a series of definitions of "the beautiful" but, rather, as an intellectual rupture from which another way of thinking about the relation between subjectivity and art is inaugurated.

From this point of view, he understands art as "a particular mode of manifestation of the spirit" (in a Hegelian sense), since here, the "spirit" is not an entity transcendent to art, but on the contrary, a form of thought inscribed in the particular rationality of the work. He thus affirms that the psychoanalytic mode of interpretation finds its conditions of inscription in an epochal horizon within which certain forms and modes of "unconscious thought" are already operating, and thus links the modes of aesthetic interpretation to psychoanalytic thought.

Already in 1900, in "The Interpretation of Dreams", Freud argues that dreams give hallucinatory form to desires, longings, and nostalgia that are interwoven with memories building fantasies. And in this sense, he provides the psychic mechanism by which the phantasy, the unconscious, flows into consciousness. In dream work, energy is coupled from one trace to another, by condensation and displacement in transferring movement. The images or visual stimuli that were first perception, are now—in a regressive sense—traces or sensorial residues and serve dreams as raw material, constructing and deconstructing images, in general, in the sense of wish fulfillment. The regard for figurability is the reason why these thoughts, memories, traces, sensations, and percepts give form to images that, transfigured from their original meaning, are subverted.

In addition, Freud argues:

> [...] It should also be remembered here that it is not only in dreams that such transformations of ideas into sensory images occur: they are also found in hallucinations and visions, which may appear as independent entities, so to say, in health or as symptoms in the psychoneuroses.
> (Freud, 1900, p. 535)

In the aesthetic experience (Goldstein, 2005) the progredient and regressive senses are superimposed in a tilting movement. The dream is not the aesthetic experience, but certain aspects of the dynamics of the dream are present in it. The time of the aesthetic experience is also the present ... and in it there is an acceleration of the images that, superimposed, unfold as in the timeless time belonging to dreams and daytime fantasies. It is an experience that admits, paradoxically, consciousness and the flow of the unconscious in the same time outside of pathology.

Freud used the works of great artists to corroborate the universality of his clinical discoveries and his theoretical models, although the angle from which he linked them with art was modified as he developed the different topics of his theory on psychic functioning. Thus, it could be assumed that there was a first period, from 1900 to 1923, in which Freud linked with art based on the model of the first topic that divided the mental apparatus into strata depending on their accessibility to consciousness. From this perspective, artistic creation was understood as the result of a special capacity of the artist to make contact with preconscious and unconscious mental contents—generally repressed sexual or aggressive impulses—and to express them, metaphorically, through the mechanisms of displacement and condensation, which allow the dreamer to disguise those repressed impulses and to satisfy them, circumventing censorship. This vision was rooted in the current of romantic literary criticism predominant in the first half of the 19th century that influenced Freud which considered artistic creativity as a form of discharge and expression of the artist's intense emotions.

At that time in Freud's work, the possibility of inferring conditions of childhood life and history in artists and linking them with the correlate of their artistic production was one of his interests, among other substantial ones. Thus, in " Leonardo Da Vinci and a Memory of his Childhood" (1910) Freud connects the characteristics of some of Leonardo's works—*La Gioconda* and the painting of *Saint Anne, the Virgin and the Child Jesus*—with aspects of his biography and character, theorizing that part of his unconscious fantasies were present in his artistic productions.

In a second theoretical moment, with the advent of the notions of Ego, Superego and Ego and its new metapsychology, the psychoanalytic understanding of artistic creation broadened and deepened: the creative process is not only an attempt to gratify repressed desires, nor simply the fruit of a special capacity of the artist to make contact with his own unconscious, but also reflects the artist's motivation to find a formal, aesthetic solution that expresses the experiences that impel him to create. The artist's personality will therefore be reflected not only in the content of the work of art—the recurring themes and symbols in his creations—but also in its formal characteristics—the form, the style with which the artist expresses his unconscious fantasies. From then on, content and form of the work of art were considered inseparable and complementary.

In this line, it is worth recalling what Freud argued in " Formulations on the Two Principles of Mental Functioning" (1911):

> Art brings about a reconciliation between the two principles in a peculiar way. An artist is originally a man who turns away from reality because he cannot come to terms with the renunciation of instinctual satisfaction which it at first demands, and who allows his erotic and ambitious wishes full play in the life of phantasy. He finds the way back to reality, however, from this world of phantasy by making use of special gifts to mould his phantasies into truths of a new kind, which are valued by men as precious reflections of reality...But he can only achieve this because other men feel the same dissatisfaction as he does with the renunciation demanded by reality, and because

> that dissatisfaction, which results from the replacement of the pleasure principle by the reality principle, is itself a part of reality.
> (p. 224)

Along these lines, Ernest Kris, an analyst who was also an art historian, in his paper entitled "Psychoanalytic Explorations of Art", argues, from this dynamic perspective, that in order to create, the artist must have sufficient ego strength and flexibility to be able to oscillate between regression and reintegration, and to allow himself what he called "regression in the service of the self": initially, the creator undergoes a temporary regression in which he makes contact with a dissociated experience that impels him to create; but then he is capable of an ego reintegration and synthesis that allows him to neutralize and sublimate the unconscious fantasy he has made contact with and express it symbolically and ambiguously through metaphors and aesthetic images, and thus differentiates artistic creation from psychotic manifestations.

On the other hand, Kris (1946) refers to the conditions for the production of the aesthetic effect of the symbol. He argues that, on the one hand, the artistic symbol must have what he calls "symbolic potential" or capacity to evoke in the audience an unconscious impact on multiple levels: for this the image has to condense the multiple unconscious aspects it contains -multiple genetic-dynamic determination, in Freud's terms, and multiple function.

Likewise, this symbol must allow the audience an "aesthetic distance", that is to say, not getting too close to the unconscious psychic reality it expresses—as it would produce repulsion or rejection—nor moving too far away from it, promoting an intellectualized defense that would prevent contact with the artistic experience.

Finally, according to Kris, the communicative intention of art has paradoxical aspects: the creator may be unconscious of his motives for creating, but the work of art—once created—has an autonomous existence and its own capacity to evoke feelings and generate thoughts that no longer depend on the author's previous intentions; the reader, the spectator, we propose, is active before the work of art and intervenes creatively with his own reading, oscillating between primary and secondary process, between regression and integration, in a process similar to that of the creator.

In this line, García Ponce (1985) synthesizes the relationship between psychoanalysis and art as follows:

> The relation of art to psychoanalysis does not consist, then, in this superficial and rhetorical illustration of psychoanalytic discoveries, but in the authentic possibility that psychoanalytic theory offers to penetrate to a certain extent into the reality of the work of art, and in turn, in the possibilities that the creator has to take from some aspects of psychoanalytic theory new points of departure for his art .... The rational acceptance of this link with the original sources, this return

> to the primitive, the infantile, in which man appears as the creator of his own myths, which is one of the most important discoveries of psychoanalysis, is presented as the vital possibility of making us masters of our own forces, as a solution for life, and therefore for art, which is always, also, life.
>
> (p. 63).

An analyzable term in relation to Freudian "estrangement" is that of *alienation* in Lacan. In the conception of the subject, Lacan (2006) creates two logical operations: alienation and separation. In Jacques Lacan's teaching there is a period in which the use of the notion of alienation is close to the Hegelian one. The "alienation there" refers to the essentially social conditions of the human world, manifested in the fact that the Imago is an effect of alienation of the self, since it is in the other that the subject locates the feeling of self, which Lacan will call "imaginary alienation".

Around 1965, in his lectures at the Di Tella Institute, Oscar Masotta (1966) saw a certain link between the estrangement of surrealism and pop-art productions. Psychoanalysis could be a way to access the mode of being of the works of both movements. The Lacanian reading of the Cartesian *cogito* ("I think where I am not and I am where I do not think") could offer, according to Masotta, a resource to account for the *pas de sens* ("passage of sense" or "without-sense", an expression that in Lacan's seminar "The Formations of the Unconscious" characterizes the operation of metaphor) with which these works were presented. The theory of the *object a* is Lacan's specific contribution to a possible aesthetics that has not necessarily been developed in depth; however, Masotta was the first to notice how prolific it was to investigate in the field of visual art with psychoanalysis as a conceptual tool, and without falling back on an applied psychoanalysis.

Eduardo Grüner (2006) stands out with his developments for an aesthetics of the *a-object*. According to the author, Grüner can make use of psychoanalysis to elucidate the visual phenomenon in logical and non-interpretive terms of works of art. Finally, within Lacanian theory, it is worth mentioning the book *Aesthetics of the pulsional* by Carlos Kuri (2015), who proposes "the irruption of the aesthetic on the conceptual distribution of psychoanalysis". Kuri elaborates the aesthetic status of subjectivity, considering its anchorage in the body and language. He argues that this aesthetic dimension is made explicit through an elucidation of the concept of drive, and is diffused in three axes: (a) the body; (b) language; and (c) sublimation.

Kuri exemplifies the impact of the aesthetic in psychoanalysis on the axis of the body with the development of "the visual", according to a reading of Freudian texts (among them, Freud's Letter 52). There the author locates the specificity of psychoanalysis as a theory of memory. However, not all elements of the psychic apparatus can be reduced to discrete mnemic components. At this point, the Greek form of catharsis is brought into relation with the first mode of the psychoanalytic method, recovering the quantitative factor involved in the perceptual pole of excitation. The next step incorporates the Lacanian theory of the imaginary, with the reference to the beautiful, to highlight the implicit drive value. From here the scheme of the Representation and the gaze, the scotoma and the schizia is made explicit, with the purpose of repositioning the sensitivity of the eye as the first aesthetic determination of the perceptual field. He indicates that Freud at this point detaches himself from the philosophical notion of representation as self-reflection, linking it to the phenomenological analyses of the late Merleau-Ponty, promoting a dimension of the body as *non-specularizable* flesh. Then, the analysis of the pictorial operation allows us to extract the drive structure of the scopic field: the "give-to-see".

Regarding the aesthetic anchoring of the body in language, Kuri affirms that "the way of instituting language ends up making us lose the specifically aesthetic problem of the body" (p. 58). According to the author, the aesthetic field highlighted by psychoanalysis cannot be captured by the signifying articulation, opening the door to an aesthetics of the name: "The name marks what vanishes from language so that the aesthetic can be constituted".

Finally, Kuri makes a detailed analysis of the theoretical problems of sublimation in Freudian terms. He argues that, beyond the notion of sublimation as a limit, as an expression of repression, it is in the separation of the sexual goal that the status of sublimation as creation intervenes: the aesthetic experience is an installer of values and, this, its performative aspect (in an aesthetics of gesture), ends up sealing the pact between sensation and the constitution of a name.

We now see the absolute relevance of psychoanalytic theory to address the notion of aesthetic experience and estrangement.

2.1.2 *Contemporary ideas on the relation between aesthetics and psychoanalysis*

Numerous current studies address from different disciplines, aesthetics, the subject-object relation, estrangement, knowledge, psychopathology, and art education.

In the field of anthropology, Alvarez Pedrosian published an article in 2009 analyzing the place of estrangement in the origins of philosophical and anthropological theories on access to knowledge. He postulates that, as an action, it has had its own weight as a strategy for the investigation of human experience. In these terms, "estrangement from reality" from a more or less marginal position, is a way of approaching practices that allows him to study some of them, social or cultural, open to new meanings outside his own "cognitive impositions". Thus, estrangement is a contradictory unity: it is approximation and distancing, it is appealing to estrangement in order to approach the phenomenon it tries to understand. What is interesting about his developments is that he focuses on the notion of estrangement in one of his definitions, which refers to the action of estrangement as a form of access and approach to the stranger in order to assimilate it to one's own and, in this process, the possibility of differentiation between the self and the stranger is raised, as recognition of otherness.

Within the field of aesthetics, but more focused on the plane of literary studies, Pedro Serra, in the article we cited in the previous chapter, takes up the notion of estrangement in relation to Russian aesthetic formalism (Serra, 2005, p.33). He proposes an essay where he reviews the notion of "estrangement" coined by Viktor Shklovski around 1917 in relation to the idea of art as artifice and links it with the concepts of "epiphany" and "late style" developed by Hans Ulrich Gumbrecht, Theodor Adorno and Edward Said, respectively, trying to characterize the complex encounter of the subject with art as a desired experience. In this work, described in depth in the background chapter, the author relates the "defamiliarization" inherent to the encounter with the object of art in the aesthetic experience with a sensitive phenomenon: the epiphany of the instant, surprise and intensity; with an alteration of the normal perception of time that places the subject in the present, but outside of it.

In his doctoral thesis, Esteban Guio Aguilar (2015) contributes to the clarification of the interpretive processes that occur in the face of what he calls the "aesthetic symbol" in order to understand aesthetic functioning. It is an approach focused on the cognitive impact of the aesthetic experience, on the promotion of a new type of knowledge based on it, which finds its central reference in Dewey's pragmatism. On the other hand, and now in the field of Education, Carlos Montenegro Ortiz published in 2014, an article entitled "Art and Aesthetic Experience", also focused on Dewey's thought, where his ideas are linked to the field of education, specifically with the artistic one. This development emphasizes the process of internalization of new knowledge (from the aesthetic experience) that arises from the individual's everyday life during which he interacts with his environment to satisfy needs and purposes. In its developments, the value of the socio-historical reading of the aesthetic experience and culture is emphasized.

On the other hand, Pablo Cabrera Pérez, in his thesis "Freud: Inquiries about the Subject, Otherness and Experience", 2015, reviews the different conceptualizations in Freud's work regarding the notion of the subject and experience, and its implications arising from changing definitions of the notion of otherness. He argues that, in his aesthetic writings on art, Freud takes up a dimension opened by Nietzsche and Marx in relation to the place of "the individual" in collective productions. It is in artistic production and in the encounter with the object of art that the subject encounters what is alien to himself, the "shadow", the "other", addressing the very complexity of the question of the dialectic between the subject and the alter-ego.

Within the psychoanalytic field, Graciela Brodsky published an article on analytic clinical work focusing on the place of surprise and its clinical value. She refers to surprise as a product of failures in the defenses, an instant where the unconscious emerges within the analytic field. She says: "Surprise that something whose original incidence was marked as trauma, as Lacan states in "*De la psychanalyse dans ses rapports avec la réalité*" ("Of psychoanalysis in its relations with reality"). Thus, he relates surprise to shock, to impact on repetitions, to the way in which the object of art bursts into spatio-temporal continuity, establishing the mark of the event. In this sense, the analyst's interpretation, according to Brodsky, must have the same psychic impact in terms of imposing a wedge in the time of repetition.

2.2 Aesthetic experience and metapsychology

To begin with, we synthesize the developments of two authors who link the notion of aesthetic experience with the process of identification and separation that occurs in the encounter with the art object and whose modality is an expression of early object relations: Melanie Klein and Hanna Segal.

These different models of internalized object relations provided new perspectives for understanding artistic creativity: according to Melanie Klein, the work of art symbolically expresses the unconscious fantasies of the *self*'s relations with its archaic internal objects and, in particular, the conflict between destructiveness and reparation towards the total object inherent to the depressive position. Hanna Segal expanded this view and added that aesthetic creativity also involves the mechanism of idealization, typical of the paranoid-schizoid position: the artist tries to create an experience in which the ideal object is felt to be part of the *self* and at the same time a separate and independent object.

In this context, Gilbert Rose argues in "Reflections on aspects of aesthetic experience from the perspective of the *rapprochement* phase" that in aesthetic experience the viewer oscillates between a feeling of fusion and temporary identification with the work of art, which allows deep contact with feelings and desires of our past and a subsequent separation and new integration of its internal and external reality; the oscillation between fusion and differentiation in the mother-baby relationship is, according to Rose, the primary antecedent of aesthetic experience.

2.2.1 *An encounter with the real: Three aesthetics in Lacan*

On the other hand, Recalcati et al. (2006) elaborates in *Lacan's Three Aesthetics* by localizing Lacan's most significant productions with respect to art. Recalcati et al. emphasizes that they are three forms of artistic creation and its product, which insist, in an unprecedented way, on placing art in a determining relationship with the real. Thus, the three aesthetics imply the turn in Lacan's work towards the real where Lacan's aesthetic interest cannot be separated from the ethics of psychoanalysis and its practice.

These are different ways of psychoanalytically defining the essence of the work of art, ways that are not mutually exclusive, but rather coexist in constant tension. Recalcati et al. also affirms that the perspective of the "three aesthetics" is Freudian, three different paradigms of jouissance are founded and implied, three different ways of implying the drive real.

These three topics are: the aesthetics of emptiness, the anamorphic aesthetics and the aesthetics of the letter. Authors refers to Lacan's seminars 7 and 11 in relation to the aesthetics of emptiness, insofar as Art is a signifying organization of a radical, extra-signifying alterity. The functioning of the unconscious is indeed structured as a language, it does have a signifying functioning, but, from *Seminar VII* onward, a dimension appears at the very center of this functioning that cannot be reduced to that of the signifier and that, thanks to this irreducibility, to this resistance, is constituted as a place (emptiness) of origin of another possible representation. Art, like the experience of psychoanalysis, neither avoids nor obstructs, but skirts the central void of the Thing. The thesis of art as "organization of the void" places the work of art in a decisive relation to the real of the Thing. The aesthetics of the void is an aesthetics of the real, an aesthetics in relation to the real, that does not degrade into a realist cult of the thing as happens in much contemporary art.

The Lacanian thesis of the work of art as the edge of *das Ding*'s void encourages us to preserve, on the contrary, an essential distance between the work of art and the void that it organizes and circumscribes. In this first aesthetic, art is defined as a symbolic practice oriented to deal with *the ungovernable excess of the real*. The beautiful as a barrier against the vortex of *das Ding* seems to return to the Freud of the poet and daydreams, where he recognizes "true poetic art" as the ability to make the repugnant and unpleasant bearable.

However, the beautiful, in order to preserve its aesthetic force, must be in relation to the real; beauty is an Apollonian veil that must make us sense the Dionysian chaos that pulsates in it, as I develop in my previous book *The Aesthetic Experience* (Goldstein, 2005). Paradoxically, the beautiful brings us closer to the Thing and yet keeps us separate from it.

There is no work of art that does not imply sublimation activity, or a mediation, a defense against the real. Hence the relationship that Lacan establishes with this first topic regarding artistic creation that Recalcati et al. describes. In *Seminar 7*, Lacan (2007) refers mainly to the apparently more everyday dimension of the object (apples, matchboxes, peasant shoes) to show the action of artistic sublimation as actions of presentification-absentification of the Thing.

In this sense, the work of art imitates the objects it represents, but only to extract a new, unprecedented, unrepresentable meaning. In this sense, the represented object is therefore not so much in relation to the object of nature, but rather in relation to the emptiness of the thing.

The second aesthetic is an anamorphic aesthetic, and has its point of condensation in *Seminar 11 (2006)*. It fundamentally theorizes art as an anamorphic encounter with the real: its criterion is not the beautiful as a symbolic barrier in our confrontations with horror (aesthetics of emptiness), but the "picture function" as a function that presentifies the unrepresentable. In this seminar, jouissance appears localized, structurally bordered, through the operation of symbolic castration that distributes it, fragmenting it, on the edges of the drive orifices of the subject's body.

Art is no longer called upon to exercise a function of organization and bordering of the real, but rather to make possible precisely the encounter with the real. It is more an aesthetics of the *tyché* than an organization of the void. The accent is no longer placed on the everyday object from which the Thing is extracted but on the anamorphic object (suspended and oblique) as that which operates an ominous rupture of the familiar.

Lacan defines an aesthetic criterion to differentiate that which is art from that which is not. There is a work of art only where the "painting function" is in action. This function has two senses: on the one hand, the object of art must have the capacity to produce an encounter with the real; the idea of apprehending the work is inverted. It is not the subject that contemplates, but the object must have the capacity to "catch" the subject. On the other hand, this "painting function" refers to a question about the figurability of the subject. Where the object of art must be able to take the subject to the "limit" of its possibility of representation. Lacan alludes to the "stain function" and argues that the stain is a function of annihilation of the subject of representation, since it shocks the being of the subject and annihilates it. There is a work of art when there is an encounter with the stain, with that which pierces the purely representative framework of the semantic organization of the work.

Finally, Lacan's third aesthetic is that of the letter. Here the real is no longer in relation to the abyss of *das Ding*, and is not even configured as a localized, partialized remainder, captured in the excess detail of the anamorphic figure. The third aesthetic is an aesthetic of singularity. At the center is the function of the painting as a *function of the letter*. The letter is the contingent encounter with that which has always been, with the essence as the "already been". It is a new theory of the encounter. In the third aesthetic a new theory of the encounter leads us to the singular dimension of the act as a modality of separation of the subject from the symbolic shadow of the Other.

Recalcati et al. is concerned with highlighting the dual status of singularity: (a) Absolutely necessary: the fall of the rain that manifests the action of the Other is absolutely necessary; and (b) Absolutely contingent: the singular imprint that cannot be reduced to an epiphenomenon of this fall—it is no longer the linear effect of a deterministic cause.

The third aesthetic presupposes a signifier loose in the chain, a non-articulation, a singular absolute eccentric to the universality of the signifier. While in the first aesthetic the irreducible excess of the real is constituted in the Thing, with art manifested as its signifying organization, in the second aesthetic this excess is all internal to the work (it is its ominous *punctum*-extimus); in the third aesthetic this is manifested in the singular, which is revealed to be marked by repetition, by the necessity of repetition, a repetition intertwined with the purest contingency. The excess of the real—irreducible to the signifier—manifests itself in the singularity of the letter as destiny.

2.2.2 *The symbolic, the relation of the unknown, and the object of perspective*

On the other hand, Rosolato, in his text *The relation of the unknown* (1978), refers to Freud's fragment on the Acropolis to advance on this "feeling of strangeness". The author links the psychoanalytic study of art with a search for truth, "circumscribing complex forms of pleasure and desire" (p. 9) and thus allowing the study of the symbolic.

Just as in several of his writings he advances on the links of the symbolic with the symbolic organization related to the father, in his theorizations on that "feeling of elation" prompted by the encounter with the art object he establishes a specific relationship between the mother and the unknown.

Rosolato says specifically in relation to Freud at the Acropolis:

> ... such a feeling of strangeness emanates from the maternal aura and the vision of the temple was the occasion to understand the movement that displaced the mother's relationship as a stranger towards a contemplation, a spiritual quest that culminates in the concern for preserving the threatened psychoanalytic discoveries
>
> (p. 11).

To argue such a relation, he links the relation of the unknown with archaic myths and the figure of the mythological mother, Mother Earth, the Night, in short, the set of "primordial mothers". Rosolato states that the relationship with the mother modulates the relationship of the unknown in reality as well as in fantasy and is determined by the possibilities of maternal desire for the father.

If the relationship with the mother is weak, he maintains, the relationship with the stranger cannot be instituted or used for pleasure; it will be forcluded, giving rise to delirium in order to obturate the anguish of emptiness. If it is too dominant, there will also be difficulties, dominated by flight. Basically, what the author argues is that the relationship with the unknown brings into play the relationship with death. And the encounter with the art object, in terms of the aesthetic experience, shows a trace of that relationship through the feeling of estrangement.

The woman occupies the central place in the dialectic between life and death according to Rosolato, referring to Freud and his analysis of "The Theme of the Three Caskets" (1913). There he elaborates on the goddesses of fertility and death and the possibilities of substitution according to desire.

Thus, he proposes three relationships between man and woman: one that enlightens him, one that accompanies him and one that destroys him.

These relationships are supported by all Eastern and Western mythology and are unconsciously played out in the place of the primordial mother.

For Rosolato (1978), the place of the unknown is always blocked in psychic systems by "the images that dictate our desires" whose purpose is to control the fear or anguish that death promotes.

In the encounter with the art object, in that state of estrangement that promotes the emergence of an ambiguous pleasure, there arises, according to Rosolato, an emergence of "old experiences of the relation with the unknown when the child tries to rediscover the object or a known pleasure and discovers the excellence of another pleasure hitherto never tasted" (Rosolato, 1978, p. 15). In this way, if the relationship with the mother is sufficiently plastic, if the maternal conditions allow it and "the lack is not too rigorous", then "the relationship with the unknown and pleasure unite, each becoming a pillar for the other and, in an exemplary way, with the aspiration to vital experiences, intellectual curiosity and epistemophilia" (p. 15).

In these terms, Rosolato is one of the most fruitful antecedents regarding the indissoluble relation between pleasure and uncertainty, between pleasure and displeasure, which promotes the encounter with the art object at the moment of aesthetic experience.

2.2.3 *Aesthetic form and the formal conditions of the mind*

Gilbert Rose, in his book *The Power of Form* (1992), proposes a view of aesthetics based on the modes of psychic functioning. He argues that artistic creation is more than an impulsive destiny, it is also, and primarily, a scenario of conflicts between "conscious and unconscious interests of the ego".

On the other hand, he affirms that the mind functions by integrating primary and secondary processes, whose relation with reality is variable. In these terms, the primary process corresponds to a perception of constant time, of space as occupied by fused objects and the person as a conglomerate of impulses tending to action. The secondary process is linked, on the other hand, to the perception of segmented time, clearly defined objects and the rational person. Thus, the modes of orientation for defining time, space and person vary and complement each other in different ways. For example, this relation is different if we are talking about dreams or a planned action.

According to the author, this complex relationship between opposing processes impacts to some extent on conceptualizations of other processes, for example, imagination. The latter could be understood adaptively as a transitional process between the self and the external world; a genetic view would pay attention to the dynamics between narcissistic fusion with the mother and movements towards separation and individuation. In summary, says Rose (1992): "We all face a dialectic between ambiguity and control: fusion vs. separation in time and space; feeling vs. thinking within the person" (p. 42).

And he postulates that "aesthetic form reflects and harmonizes the discrepancies and tensions originating in the formal characteristics of the mind … it sharpens thought and feeling, separation and fusion" (p. 42).

In this way, this author is a fundamental antecedent, not only because he proposes a way of approaching the work of art from an unconscious mind, from an unconscious conflict, but also because he affirms that it is this same dynamic that is stimulated by the work of art.

2.3 Psychic structuring and the dialectic of subject/object and self/non-self

2.3.1 *The dialectics of the subject/object and self/non-self relationship in the aesthetic experience*

There are various forms of memory in art, memory that constitutes and inhabits the soul of the art object that, as a symbolic construct, is embodied in the work. It is that which overflows its autonomy, making the effect of subject in the other. This effect is constituted in experience, and approaches another type of knowledge, related to the knowledge of oneself, showing the dialectical function of alienation and separation of the I/not-I. In this dialectic, a moment of the self is the moment when the other is the subject of the work of art. In that dialectic, a particular moment of aesthetic experience, there is the appropriation of something of the lost memory, the strange, the unknown. Now, it is also in that dialectic, which is perceived as "depersonalization" or "foreignness"—in Freudian terms—where the state of estrangement occurs.

There are multiple references within psychoanalysis regarding the indissoluble and paradoxical link between the subject and the object, between the self and the foreign, between the known and the strange. Winnicott and his transitional thinking is one of the theoretical pillars.

Winnicott places the "origin" of the *other* within the framework of early infancy and the first moments of the mother-baby relationship. The maternal disposition to shelter and sustain her baby, the desire to be required and the deep identification (conscious and unconscious) in absolute dependence, moves the mother to produce and sustain a situation that becomes the origin of the emergence of an external object for her baby. Winnicott called this unprecedented situation "first (feeding) theoretical lactation", a moment of "primary psychic creation" (Winnicott, 1988, p. 106).

The baby feels instinctive and pressing needs accompanied by predatory ideas. The mother possesses the breast and the faculty to produce its nourishment. These two phenomena do not establish a mutual relationship until mother and child live and feel together. Being mature and physically capable, the mother is the one who must be tolerant and understanding so that she is the one who produces a situation that hopefully can become the first link between the little one and an external object (Winnicott, 1999, p. 209).

Thus, in this essential encounter between mother and baby, based on their mutual inherent inequality, the primary relationship that the baby establishes with external reality is cemented in moments of encounter and illusion in which a fragment of the baby's experience comes to be considered a thing belonging to external reality or a hallucination.

It thus refers to a point of passage between something that begins in the register of a vague bodily sensation of discomfort (hunger) that requires relief, and the emergence of something existing outside the *self* that is just what is required to calm down. There is something in the order of omnipotence that becomes effective in the baby's experience and makes present the paradox of helplessness-omnipotence, and that of creation-finding. There is also something paradoxical in the mutuality of experience that Winnicott describes. There is a necessary complementarity between the baby's experience and the mother's adaptive behavior.

In line with his proposal of paradoxical tensions to think about the subject's relationship with the external world, to review the subject-object and own-alien relationship; Winnicott proposes, in 1951, a hypothesis that he reworks in 1971, regarding the existence of the object and transitional phenomena. In doing so, he opens an area of theoretical and clinical richness.

The idea that the transitional object is a form of objects of use makes it possible to include a thirdness. It is *between* the mother and the child that this particular type of use object appears: neither fully objective nor subjective. This object and these transitional phenomena belong to an intermediate zone of experience (between the thumb and the teddy bear, between oral eroticism and the object relation), between the internal, subjective and reserved reality and external reality, the objectively perceived and therefore shareable. This intermediate zone of experience, neither inside nor outside, becomes the "third zone" or potential space, where personal creativity unfolds, making these objects emerge, just as it later does in play and in cultural phenomena. What is the nature of the transitional object? It is not an internal object, nor an external object, it is at the limit, neither inside nor outside, and it serves to connect, unite and separate these zones at the same time. It is accessed through contact with the senses, it is visible, palpable, and the child exercises omnipotent dominion over it, dominion by manipulation, based on the pleasure of coordination and muscular eroticism. It is a possession, the first non-I possession. This marks its function, aiming at separation. It is a possession (it belongs to me; therefore, it is not I) for the child, it is his creation, but it was already in the world waiting to be found, an essential paradox to respect and not to impoverish by asking whether it was created or found. The transitional object "inaugurates an affectionate type of relationship with the object", says Winnicott in *Reality and Play*, in 1971, which in a certain way distances us from the Freudian and Kleinian drives, and enables transit through the idea of separation from the mother, her failures, her absence. It is this conjunction of absence, mitigated by the tangible presence of the transitional object, at the same time that it is recognized as absence, which is the driving force of the introduction to symbolization.

In solidarity with the above, it can be affirmed that play, or rather playing, is the keystone of his thinking: "In play, and only in play, can the child or adult create and use the whole personality; the individual discovers his *self* only when he shows himself to be a creator", asserts Winnicott (1971, p. 80). For him, play is situated in the intermediate area of transitional phenomena that determine cultural experience. In this sense, Winnicott conceives play as a space of production *per se*. Cultural experience, art, and its specificity condensed in the art object is a direct extension of play and determines the occurrence of aesthetic experience. It arises in the potential space between external reality or *shared reality* and internal reality. Cultural experience implies accepting tradition and assuming the established, in order to question it with a new way of *creating the world*. The transitional therefore alludes to a particular mode of use of the object because it supposes both the external and the internal.

On the other hand, for Winnicott (1971) as for Aulagnier (1977), a paradox is present in the origins of psychic life: the *infant*'s experience promotes reactions in the other, even when this other is unknown to him; but this experience is only such in function of what it promotes in the other. A general statement can then be constructed: the object exists psychically by virtue of its power to modify the sensory response and thus acts on psychic experience. However, what is external to the psyche only exists if it supports investiture. The parents, as representatives of the external world, contribute to the *infant*'s state of completeness, a state that is part of the pictographic representation: complementary object-zone. In some sense, the work of art, the object of art, impacts on this plane of representation.

In fact, in 1977, Aulagnier advances this idea by giving the subject-object a "plus" to be added to this complementarity. The plus-zone of the complementary object is thus proposed, where different obstacles in the process of psychic constitution are elaborated (the child's own failures, the constitutional amount of death drive, environmental failure, etc.).

The elements that constitute the complementary object-zone, placed in relation by the pictogram, are inseparable. The image of the bodily thing, that plus of the object in the complementary zone, is a production with a quality of certainty, a quality that characterizes the pictogram and is anchored in the body-world as representative of the non-repressed, beyond the primary process. This affirmation supports the hypothesis that the aesthetic experience as an encounter with the art object promotes creative processes anchored in the pictogram as a sensorial production with somatic quality, beyond the encounter with the repressed - as shown below.

Green joins Aulagnier's approach when he places this concept of "representative" in a *space prior* to that of "signifier", a position that in both authors accounts for a different model of psychic construction (Green, 1995).

Aulagnier also investigates the relation between the organization of psychic space, of somatic space and of the psychic environment. In this sense, he clearly proposes a necessary dialectic between the subject and the object in which they mutually constitute each other.

In this way, it is articulated with Freudian approaches where the psychic environment, of which both Winnicott and Aulagnier speak, is described as the object of the specific and adequate action: the experienced individual who provides nourishment and approaches as a sexual object in a favorable position; under these conditions, the experience of satisfaction is inscribed as an *event* in the psyche. I underline this term, "event", already used by Freud, in order to emphasize its relation with what Aulagnier formulated: the "theory of the encounter", to which she assigns a primordial role.

In structural and no longer intersubjective terms, Lacan expresses his thinking on the transitional in relation to anguish. Here the transitional object is a response to a trauma of origin that has to do with the fact that human reality is a reality of language and consequently with the denaturalization of instinct. The reading of the transitional object as ceasable anticipates in Lacan the character of the *object a.* According to Vázquez (2007) for Lacan, Winnicott gives the transitional object this function of a ceasable object like a torn piece, a corner of a blanket, a pacifier. She argues that the subject consoles himself and at the same time allows the replacement of the natural object and open ways to metonymy.

This statement maintains a profound relation with reflections possible when investigating the aesthetic experience. Pabello and Romero (2006) argue that analyzing the aesthetic experience and art as creation brings with it a way of approaching the world, since outside the margins imposed on it as knowledge of reality, *the rules that define what is known are disrupted and transcend the sphere of the knowable*, creating their own rules. Paradoxical thinking is evident, according to these authors, given that reflection on art itself implies, at the same time, the concurrence of two almost opposite thoughts: on the one hand, a moment of "synthesis" in the expression and resolution of experience (experience with meaning) and, on the other, a kind of escape or "vanishing point" related to the notions of sublimation, fantasy, delirium or unreality related to the attempt to conceptualize the state of estrangement inherent to the aesthetic experience. A state where new associations and correspondences are promoted. The forms of "knowledge" that involve the encounter with art and engage the subject emerge as "truth" in the "unconscious memory". This is produced through the normativity of art itself, which is non-discursive letter and manifests itself as a form of sensibility, which constitutes the aesthetic experience, which is metaphor and metonymy, and condition of its poetics.

This seems to be a central point of aesthetic experience: it is the alienating moment of experience itself, a state of estrangement of the subject in relation to itself and/or in relation to what is perceived. Alienating truth in which the self is not unique and coherent, since to its very vigilant consciousness ascends a reality that deceives it ... by admitting the split, it admits that I am also another (*car je est un autre*, in Rimbaud's words). The other becomes me and the me becomes alienated in the other, showing the dialectical function of alienation and separation of the me/not-me from the times of identification jubilation, where the foundations of our aesthetic possibility reside, where we see ourselves and where we are looked at.

A modality of *dialectical splitting* is then established, understood as structuring the admission of doubt, as split consciousness, where the denial sustained in the non-pathological aspects of feelings of alienation is throwing onto ourselves the possibility of the aesthetic experience. Both are part of the same thing; the splitting of the self and alienation, give rise to experience, admitting the irruption of the unconscious into intended consciousness.

The same dialectic and indissoluble relation between subject and object, between self and non-self, promotes the question: what is the place or category where the object of art is situated? The aforementioned allows us to define it from a modern object category, situated in a transitional place. As an object of aesthetic experience, it inhabits an intermediate zone, a zone of the potentiality of culture. The possibility of inhabiting an intermediate place commits it to a momentary fusion, where an instant lasts a thousand years and the limits of reality and fantasy merge and "blur". A place where" integrating fusion" takes place, which is, at the same time, the source of pleasure of this experience.

These phenomena—the aesthetic phenomena—are produced in a topic, a target *place* in the space of culture. Winnicott, in *Reality and Play*, says: "But the phenomena that possess reality in the zone whose existence I postulate belong to the experience of the relationship with objects [...] characteristic, for example, of two people in love" (Winnicott, 1971, p. 132).

Transference, infatuation, condition of the aesthetic experience in the actuality of desire, whose character is enabled, also according to Gilbert Rose, by the "necessary illusion" that covers the experience and is part of this encounter.

Estrangement already implies the beginning of the encounter with another by estranging us in another, giving rise to an experience that, as has been said, we could call "on the edge". Thus, this experience as an edge prior to fusion is part of an indissoluble dialectical condition.

Aesthetic experience as an experience on the edge places us on a threshold, the "threshold of perception", where the differences between reason and sensation are erased. This experience is possible when it is symbolically sustained by the subject of the experience, a necessary condition for the edge not to be too disturbing ... as in the presence of a hole that is not in the object, but the unfolding of an emptiness of experience in the very self of the emptied subject. Following Kris (1946), the object must summon that edge precisely in a way to promote that ambiguity, that necessary confusion, without it having an impact triggering a defensive response. That virtual edge that is crossed, the edge of the difference or limit between subject and object, implies the admission of a sensory shock that, by crossing the educated shell of the ego armor of reality, reaches the emotion of a symbolized subject.

Coinciding with Agamben's description of the place of aesthetic experience, one could say, in the author's words, that it is in that place situated between narcissistic love and external object choice that the creations of human culture can be placed (Goldstein, 2005).

And Winnicott states:

> The place of cultural experience is the potential space that exists between the individual and the environment, times of the first experiences that exist there between the subjective object and the objectively perceived object, between the extensions of the self and the not-self.
>
> (p. 26).

He then conceptualizes what he called "the third zone", that of cultural experience, which is a derivative of play. In that zone, as neutral territory, there is "relief" from the tension imposed by the "never-ending task of the acceptance of reality, the eternal human task of linking inner and outer reality."

> Suspension of the tensions that produce relief, and overlapping of the common experience, as happens in the experiences in philosophy, in religion and in art. And even more, I would say, the gain of pleasure emerges as a promise produced by the encounter with the object of art, in the plus of pleasure transferred by the artist himself when realizing the work.
>
> (Winnicott, 1971, p. 41).

The aesthetic experience *is an* event, a condition of mediation that in turn is an encounter that combines in its consummation the close experience of the felt past with the immediate present, actualizing a type of sensual attention, different from that of a drive seeking discharge. "Time, space and person re-fuse and re-form restoring an enriched balance in complexity," asserts Rose in *The Power of Aesthetic Form*. The "controlled ambiguity", as on the Acropolis, would be the key that allows a gain of pleasure, inherent to aesthetic pleasure, similar to previous pleasure, close to the idea of sublimation, the idea of non-discharge by means of processes inherent to this experience, such as the tertiary processes. The aesthetic experience is intimately related to "the apprehension of beauty", which in the midst of "a certain overwhelming sensation" produces a network of identifications through which one is dragged, according to Meltzer and Harris Williams (1990), as if between fluid limits and vanishing edges, a sort of "enveloping spell", a dream evoked and contained that, in coming and going, finds its symbolic form.

2.4 Fantasy, "Thinking sensation" and symbolization: Artistic creation

"Artists are violent, alienated beings."

Mc Dougall, J. et al. (2010).

In 1908 and 1911, respectively, Freud published, "The Creative Writers and Day-dreaming" and "Formulations on the Two Principles of Mental Functioning". In these texts, Freud argues that the source of the poet's creative activity lies in daydreams or fantasies, which are in adults a substitute for children's play. Here fantasizing is understood as an activity that acquires autonomous deployment when the principle of reality is established to the extent that it is not subjected to its conditions of functioning. Equaling creative thinking to fantasizing, it can be affirmed that it is a type of thinking at the service of wish fulfillment that inhibits reality judging, knowledge and rational thought.

In these texts, reality is connoted as a frustrating element that must be denied, disguised, distorted, and therefore the object of art seeks to somehow circumvent the restrictive imprint of reality. In dreaming and daydreaming we find desire as a motor and its objects will be the objects of desire that are figured. This implies a difference with respect to the aesthetic experience, where we are dealing with a created object. That object which, as a human *construct*, is expropriated from subjectivity, belongs to cultural reality. It is an object transferred from *cathexis* that, as a seductive object, invites us to a process of fusion as a primordial object of love.

In other Freudian texts, fantasies are no longer at the service of avoiding the frustration of reality but are defensive constructions in relation to ethical or aesthetic norms to avoid the recognition of incestuous desire. It is no longer a matter of the avoidance of reality but of the contradiction between desires and the requirements of the ideals resulting from post-oedipal identifications. As a product, fantasy expresses the mechanism of "cooperation" between the unconscious and the preconscious, which is opposed to repression at the level of the link between representations. Repression stabilizes the gap between the two systems and cooperation attempts to bridge the gap through phantasies and other products (Freud, 1911). The phantasy acts as a point of union, bringing thing and word representations closer together, reaching an imaginary staging where desire is consolidated by circumventing repression. The visual elements of the thing representations selectively organize word representations. Thus, the constitutive elements of fantasy are the perceptual (seen and experienced), the heard (the parents' words), the drive articulated in desiring motions, and the singular oedipal significations (Freud, 1908).

Thus, fantasy is not defined in opposition to reality but constitutes a transactional formation between various intrapsychic instances and processes. Piera Aulagnier (1997) conceptualizes the *narcissistic contract* as the pact through which the subject invests identification positions in social discourse and commits to formulating the fundamental statements of the group of origin. The social space is the one to which the subject comes and offers himself, the psychic organizer that enables the distance from the primary invested objects, offering himself as a support of ideals and identificatory emblems mediated by the relations with those first objects. In this sense, Aulagnier (1997) argues that the psyche and the world are born as a result of a "state of encounter", arising from several mis-encounters, non-encounters, encounters, and re-encounters. The author calls it the state of existent, that is to say, the state of whatever is maintained in psychic life, understood as the survival of the body, the support of a libidinal investiture that dominates the action of Thanatos. It is in this movement of binding, unbinding, and rebinding that the psyche is constituted by means of the earliest identifications.

What is relevant is that this relationship determines a relational field between subject and subject, a field in which the world of possible exchanges is defined. Associations and traces work in a continuous process of bonding before the perception of that which the object provokes in the aesthetic experience and, in the case of bonding, allows, in my understanding, the "apprehension of beauty", a term coined by Meltzer and Harris Williams (1990). In the case of an impossible ligature, the anxiety signal warns us that the beautiful is threatening.

As Freud maintains in "The Uncanny" (1919, p. 243), certain feared objects or fantasies are nothing more than a transmutation that carries not terror, but a certain concupiscence: "the fantasy of living in the mother's womb". The mother is also undoubtedly an overwhelming object, a beloved primordial object of psychoanalysis and art, once and a thousand times sought after as a longed-for, lost and represented object. The object of aesthetic experience awaits us and then captures us, for that is precisely the place of aesthetic experience, the place of capture, the place that subsumes us and deceives us in its perfect, almost human imperfection. In the Parthenon, was Freud so far from romantic evocation? Lost and enraptured, he seemed to falter at the sight of the Acropolis. There was something in the landscape that, like a screen memory, did not seem to "fit". And it is in front of that monument, a paradox transformed from matter to illusion, from movement to experience, that the alienated man believes he loses consciousness.

The references to the fantasies evoked by the effect of the aesthetic experience link the impact of the ambiguous object with the mobilization of the unconscious in terms of effects on narcissism.

In the storytelling of the "disturbance" at the Acropolis, both the symbolic and the sensory configure an experience in which the transferences drag the visitor, abyssed, back to the ancient times he thought forgotten. From a Lacanian perspective, these productions have a special effect on the spectator. Nasio (1994) speaks of "forms and images endowed with a singular efficacy, treated in the manner of our narcissistic unconscious self".

For this author, the imaginary and narcissistic object is a condensation of the drive force, the narcissism of the creator, and the finished form of the work of art, and therefore arouses emotion and fascination in the spectator (pp. 117–118).

Similarly, Green (1995) refers to trans-narcissistic objects. The trans-narcissistic object is a binding and potential object located between two subjects (the creator and the spectator), acting as a mediator for both unconsciouses and allowing joint or individual movements of union and separation. In this sense, and by means of the link with words or other symbols, the trans-narcissistic object would be constituted by preconscious elements of both subjects, between the projected and the introjected, between the found and the re-created, allowing communication from unconscious to unconscious through a common code, analogous to what happened in the past between the child and the mother. In each case—theater, rite, game, analysis—the trans-narcissistic object is constituted by the doubles of two absent objects, according to Green. In this way, we find the two rigorously absent and the trans-narcissistic object, *unique for each subject* that unites and separates it from the other. Objects of art necessarily fulfill this condition of trans-narcissistic objects, of singular efficacy, which puts in contact two unconsciouses, in reference to the creator of the work and the spectator. It is true that the aesthetic experience does not always take place in front of a work of art; it may be another type of stimulus. However, there are "gifted" objects that summon and have a greater potential to promote a disturbing, moving impact on the subject, as a prelude to the state of estrangement, as the knot of the aesthetic experience. The aesthetic experience is an experience with an object that has its own characteristics.

Estrangement, as a psychic state—we understand psychic in the sense given by Freud—, that is, of the soul (*Psyché* in Greek), something that is not yet formalized or metabolized, or "thought" in terms of reason, is considered a necessary state for the condition of possibility of the aesthetic experience, and it is produced from the encounter with the object of art. That encounter, between the subject of the experience and the object of art, is in the order of the event: something unexpected happens in that encounter that initiates estrangement. This encounter-event that initiates estrangement moves something physical. It is a disruptive event, insofar as there is a break or discontinuity in lived experience and in time, outside of pathology, which produces something new. It is, therefore, a non-traumatogenic disruptive event that potentially promotes metabolization, only inferable in a *posteriori* (Benyakar, 2000). Therefore, estrangement is the effect of the encounter with art as an event.

On the other hand, estrangement is a temporary state that manifests itself as a non-pathological but diffuse unreality, with blurred edges, that implies openness to the unknown, to the strange and to the intensity of the senses; it circulates in the midst of a "fluid reality" in direct relation to temporal perception. This state promotes affects that become thinkable in "a second moment", since a form of "sensible thought" is produced after a first impression, which has to do with pleasure or surprise and shock. These are diverse modes of pleasure, which is why it was called "paradoxical pleasure"; it is the affective correlate of estrangement. In the aesthetic experience, as we define it, the Dionysian and the Apollonian, pleasure, and a pleasant pain such as nostalgia, *nostos,* or something disturbing (the disturbing strangeness) that underpins the notion of paradoxical pleasure, converge in different ways. Creative processes are the way of interweaving the relationship between subject and object, between reality and fantasy, between the intrapsychic and what circulates between the self and the Other.

In the space of estrangement, the full potency of unconscious poetics emerges in an activity, as Freud says in "The Creative Writers and the Day-dreaming" (1908), akin to poeticizing; it is a mode of bonding that admits the principle of reality and the principle of pleasure, as well as and at the same time as poetic estrangement. Estrangement accounts for a situation in which the subject is the subject of the experience, involved in it, participating in an experience with the object of art, which is "transformed", or appears, accounting for its enigmatic condition. In turn, the subject is summoned to its creative potential, since the unconscious circulates in estrangement. It also gives rise to transformative potentiality as creativity. What is at stake is what configures this encounter as a space "between", a middle point of virtual encounter related to the intermediate space conceptualized by Winnicott (1971), the place of the first instant of "illusion", of the "creative gesture", genesis of the place of culture. It is in this indeterminate territory where the unexpected encounter between subject and object takes place, an asymptotic and, at the same time, alienating encounter where the condition of possibility of art objects as objects of culture resides, whose imperceptible thirdness makes the aesthetic experience a poetic estrangement.

In other words, this *encounter*, characterized as a triadic object, where the subject, the object and the field that contains them are conceived, is compatible with what is defined as "complex objects", a quality of psychoanalytic objects par excellence, as considered by Rodriguez Zoya and Aguirre (2011). This link between subject and object in the field that contains them as a "complex field" (Goldstein), "dynamic analytic field" (Baranger & Baranger, 1988), is what also interdefines their terms. It is impossible, in this case, to think of the art-object without referring to the subject and vice versa. On the other hand, in meta-psychological terms, the characteristics of this encounter, as estrangement, refer to the "impossible" encounter with the *lost object*. An object loved, feared, dreamed of, of which only something remains, either of it or of what causes it, or more complexly of its new coordinates, which "appear" where it emerges. The object of art, in its enigmatic character, as familiar as it is strange, is rediscovered. In this way something of the lost traces of pleasure and of the lost (traumatic) is recovered, in the instant of the encounter, although in a different way, as something new in the strangeness of estrangement and in the aesthetic pleasure; this is a way to go back over traces of a lost pleasure, that of the object, the other, and the possibility of affects and effects is relaunched, resonating in the sensation of being. To exist, to live of oneself.

Franco Berardi, in 2021, asked how to re-subjectivize ourselves in the face of the advance of fascism, said that "it is the task of philosophy, but **above all of psychoanalysis and of art, of poetry**" (2021).

2.5 Estrangement and subjectivation in psychoanalytic theory

The term "estrangement" refers, on the one hand, to the action of estranging or being estranged and, on the other, to the effect of estranging or being estranged, according to Ferrater Mora (2000). This dual definition is very interesting since it synthesizes the indissoluble sides of estrangement. On the one hand, the act of estrangement, linked to an instant in which the strangeness of the subject occurs with respect to himself, to that which he contemplates and to the temporal dimension in which this event takes place. On the other hand, the object that provokes an effect of estrangement, the object of art, the work of art, which has particular qualities because it can promote that state of estrangement.

Beyond his specific writings where a Freudian "aesthetic thought" can be inferred, Freud makes a first reference, in that sense, to *estrangement*, as we said, as a consequence of the subject's encounter with the art object in his letter to Rolland, where he describes what he calls a "disturbance of memory" on the Acropolis.

The Parthenon on the Acropolis was designed by the architects Ictinus and Callicrates together with the sculptor Phidias, commissioned by Pericles, explains Bellucci (in Goldstein, 2005). In honor of the goddess Athena, protector of the city, the temple was built with the most elaborate resources of the time, which, through the planning of optical effects, deceives the viewer with precise and subtle proportions. The Doric order gives its sought-after harmony by means of contradictions in the face of the pretended classical reason. This elaboration of visual effects is achieved with the "paradoxical" design that resolves aesthetic conflicts with curvatures, instead of straight lines, and progressive elongations or inclinations. A perfectly premeditated geometry gives grace and vitality to the whole, building its humanistic condition. Introducing "controlled distortions" is the "secret" key where the "exciting" dimension of the genius of ancient Greece resides. According to Bellucci, therein lies the "fusion" of the arts resolved in an integrating experience beautifully enunciated by German Romanticism, saying that, for the Greeks, the Acropolis "sang at sunset" (Belucci, in Goldstein, 2005).

In the manner of a short story, Freud relates, in an almost vertiginous tone, a trip to Athens, almost unexpectedly and with Corfu as the original destination. This sudden change is taken by Freud as something quite natural, but he admits: "It was very strange, this behavior [...] What I see there is not really real", while at the same time he doubts the existence of what he sees. He adds, referring to a sense of disbelief:

> "I stood on the Acropolis and cast my eyes around upon the landscape, a surprising thought suddenly entered my mind" (p. 224) ... a sense of some feeling of the unbelievable and the unreal in the situation at the moment. The situation included myself, the Acropolis and my perception of it" (Freud, 1936, p. 224)

Well, this incredulity, this doubt in a fragment of reality, is displaced in the utterance in two ways: first, it is referred to the past and, second, it is transferred from my presence in the Acropolis to the existence of the Acropolis itself. Thus something is produced that is equivalent to asserting that I have once doubted the real existence of the Acropolis, something that my memory disavows as incorrect, and even as impossible.

Freud theorizes, trying to clarify the feeling of confusion, about feeling of alienation (*Entfremdungsgefüh*) and says "I tried to defend myself against it, and I succeeded at the cost of a false statement about the past"; this disbelief as a disfigurement occurring on an element of objective reality... "are still little understood. They are spoken of as 'sensations', but they are obviously complicated processes, attached to particular mental contents and bound up with decisions made about those contents" (p. 245). These may arise in certain mental diseases, but are not unknown among healthy people, just as hallucinations.

In the same paper, he defines these feelings as "sensations", the product of complex processes, frequent in certain psychic illnesses, which, like "occasional hallucinations", are "failed operations of abnormal construction" like dreams. Thus, he attributes anomalous characteristics to them and also the possibility of appearing regularly in the psychic life of "healthy" people.

He refers to this sensation of estrangement from reality in the sense that, in those particular encounters with the art object, the subject may feel alien or strange to the perceived reality or may himself feel strange or "depersonalized", as we said before. He also alludes to a third possibility, its "positive counterparts," as another form of mirage.

In this way, Freud enunciates the characteristics he identifies as central to these sensations of estrangement produced in the encounter with the art object, but refuses to further deepen his theorization. However, he manages to infer that a first reading links this depersonalization with certain defense mechanisms in which repression imposes a disfigurement on memory. Then, he overturns his own associations, related to his oedipal history, where he finds the cause of the obturation of the memory.

Freud advances in his analysis of this event along three lines of thought, which I analyzed in depth in a previous paper (Goldstein, 2005); first of all, the feeling of guilt and "those who fail to succeed", both on the conceptual axis: Oedipus-repression, guilt, and parricide. This is the central path that Freud chooses to delimit the field of analysis of the "little experience", then introduces, incipiently, the problem of the ego and defense mechanisms. He only announces this theme, saying that his daughter Anna is dealing with it in her book. Finally, he advances on the problem of the feeling of alienation, opening spaces in disturbing, overlapping zones, but decides to "forbid himself to continue elucidating", as he himself expresses later, "to go so far".

This last line contains the germ of what Rancière (2009) calls "the intellectual rupture" promoted by psychoanalytic thought in relation to aesthetics, since it would be defined as paradoxical thought whose example is aesthetic interpretation but which floods the entire development of the theory. The presence of pagan abandonment is revealed in the formula of *Pathos* as an emotion that contains *something* of the non-integrated. It is in this very distant and ambiguous place of memory that the "aesthetic regime of art" defined by Rancière is constituted. In this regime, I understand, there is dynamic tension that asks not to be resolved—like Winnicott's paradox—in order to maintain the eternal contest between the Dionysian and the Apollonian and the existence of a certain relationship between thought and non-thought, Rancière affirms (2009). From the dark and enigmatic of unconscious desire emerge passions that, beyond the Apollonian, become effective in the most tremendous Dionysian overflow. There the horrors of a de-juxtaposed drive emerge, emptied and transfigured into cruelty, justified, by the *manifesto* of naturalized horror. This thesis implies a higher level of theoretical articulation on that Freudian affirmation from which, the "perception of the beautiful", summons something of the hidden, of the enigmatic inherent to the manifestation of unconscious desire, which is the sensorial support of the state of estrangement that is described and theorized about.

By way of synthesis, it is assumed that estrangement is an effect of the encounter with the object of art. That this object contains particular conditions of summoning unconscious aspects, as Kris and Freud point out, when the latter refers to the "mnemic treasure" of the Ego. This state of estrangement is a transitory psychic state, as described by Freud, outside the framework of pathology and, as we propose, *the knot or neuralgic point of aesthetic experience, in fact, is what causes it.* It should be clarified that this involves a substantial difference from the Freudian approach in that it is not only a sensation, but also the generalities of a particular psychic state and that, as a psychic state, it evidently alludes to complex processes that, on the one hand, imply a defense or denial of reality—through the state of alienation or disbelief—but, at the same time, since it touches the unconscious, promotes the unfolding of creative processes.

Thus, estrangement, as a condition of possibility of the aesthetic experience, takes place in a dynamic space of the relationship between subject and object, necessarily promotes ambiguous affects—as it allows the emergence of the ominous—and is experienced in an instant that constitutes a discontinuity in space-time perception, which gives it the character of an event.

References

Álvarez Pedrosian, E. (2009) La experiencia del extrañamiento. Artículo presentado en la VIII Reunión de Antropología del Mercosur (RAM): Diversidad y Poder en América Latina, Buenos Aires, 29 de septiembre al 2 de octubre de 2009.

Aulagnier, P. (1997/1977) La violencia de la interpretación; del pictograma al Enunciado, Buenos Aires, Amorrortu.

Baranger, M., Baranger, W. & Mom, J. M. (1988) The Infantile Psychic Trauma from us to Freud: Pure Trauma, Retroactivity and Reconstruction. International Journal Psychoanalysis, 69, 113–128.

Baumgarten, A. G. (1735) Meditationes philosophicae de nonnullis ad poema pertinentibus, quas amplissimi philosophorum ordinis consensu [Some poem-related philosophical meditations], Halle an der Saale, Johann Heinrich Grunert.

Benyakar, M. (2000) "Lo traumático y lo ominoso". Cuestionamientos Teórico-Clínicos acerca del procesamiento de las amenazas. Simposio Preparatorio de las Jornadas Trauma – Duelo – Cuerpo. Dpto. de Niños y Psicosomática. Asociación Psicoanalítica Argentina (A.P.A.) 23 de Mayo del 2000

Berardi, F. (2021) Ñ Magazine, Saturday, July 17. Buenos Aires, Editorial Clarín.

Cabrera Perez, P. (2015) "Freud: indagaciones en torno al sujeto, la alteridad y la experiencia". Tesis de postgrado. Facultad de Artes, Escuela de Posgrado, Universidad de Chile. https://repositorio.uchile.cl/bitstream/handle/2250/136743/freud-indagaciones-en-torno.pdf?sequence=1&isAllowed=y

Ferrater Mora, J. (2000) Diccionario de filosofía, Barcelona, Ariel, 4 vols.

Freud, S. (1900) "The Interpretation of Dreams". The Standard Edition of the Complete Psychological Works of Sigmund Freud, London, Hogarth Press and the Institute of Psycho-Analysis.

Freud, S. (1908) "Creative Writers and Day-Dreaming". The Standard Edition of the Complete Psychological Works of Sigmund Freud, London, Hogarth Press and the Institute of Psycho-Analysis, pp. 141–154.

Freud, S. (1910) "Leonardo Da Vinci and a Memory of his Childhood". The Standard Edition of the Complete Psychological Works of Sigmund Freud, London, Hogarth Press and the Institute of Psycho-Analysis, pp. 57–138.

Freud, S. (1911) "Formulations on the Two Principles of Mental Functioning". The Standard Edition of the Complete Psychological Works of Sigmund Freud, London, Hogarth Press and the Institute of Psycho-Analysis, pp. 213–226.

Freud, S. (1913) "The Theme of the Three Caskets". The Standard Edition of the Complete Psychological Works of Sigmund Freud, London, Hogarth Press and the Institute of Psycho-Analysis, pp. 289–302.

Freud, S. (1919) "The 'Uncanny'". The Standard Edition of the Complete Psychological Works of Sigmund Freud, London, Hogarth Press and the Institute of Psycho-Analysis, pp. 217–256.

Freud, S. (1936) "A Disturbance of Memory on the Acropolis", The Standard Edition of the Complete Psychological Works of Sigmund Freud, London, Hogarth Press and the Institute of Psycho-Analysis, pp. 237–248.

García Ponce, J. (1985) Arte y Psychoanalisis. Revista de la Universidad de México. https://www.revistadelauniversidad.mx/articles/cf144565-451b-4140-8e2d-fe17066cb5dc/arte-y-psicoanalisis
Goldstein, G. (2005) La experiencia estética, Buenos Aires, del estante editorial.
Green, A. (1995) La metapsicologia revisitada, Buenos Aires, Editorial Eudeba.
Grüner, L. E. (2006) "El Otro Imposible, entre el arte y la política", en VVAA: Jean Paul Sartre, Actualidad de un Pensamiento, Buenos Aires, Colihue.
Guio Aguilar, E. (2015) Del arte a la experiencia estética Interpretación y efectos cognitivos en la función estética. Tesis Doctoral, UNMdP.
Kris, E. (1946) Freudianism and the Literary Mind: By Frederick J. Hoffman. Baton Rouge: Louisiana State University Press, 1945.
Kuri, C. (2015) Estética de lo pulsional. Lazo y exclusión entre psicoanálisis y arte, Letra Viva, 336 págs.
Lacan, J. (2006) "El sujeto y el otro: la alienación", en El seminario de Jacques Lacan. Libro 11, Los cuatro conceptos fundamentales del psicoanálisis, cap. XVI. Buenos Aires, Paidós.
Lacan, J. (2007) La ética del psicoanálisis, El Seminario, Libro 7, (1959–1960), Buenos Aires, Paidós.
Masotta, O. (1966) Arte pop y Semántica. Dos conferencias pronunciadas en el Instituto Torcuato di Tella (1965). Centro de Artes Visuales Instituto Torcuato Di Tella; Documentos de trabajo. Segunda Edición.
McDougall, J., André, J., De M'Uzan, M., Marinov, VI, Porret, Ph., Scheneider, M., and Suchet, D. (2010) The Artist and Psychoanalysis, Serie Claves, Buenos Aires, Nueva Visión.
Meltzer, D. & Harris, M. (1988/1990) La Aprehensión de la Belleza, Buenos Aires, Spatia ed.
Montenegro Ortíz, C. (2014) Arte y experiencia estética: John Dewey. Revista nodo N° 17, 9, 95–105.
Nasio, J. D. (1994) "El magnífico niño del Psicoanálisis", in El concepto de sujeto y objeto en la teoría de Jacques Lacan, Barcelona, Gedisa.
Pabello, G. M. & Romero, V. M. A. (2006) Revista Casa del tiempo, April, 87 (07), Mexico.
Ranciere, J. (2009) The Aesthetic Unconscious, Translated by Debra Keates and James Swenson, Polity, Cambridge
Ranciere, J. (2013) Aisthesis, escenas del régimen estético del arte, Buenos Aires, Ed Manantial.
Recalcati, M., Brousse, M-H., Wajcman, G., Coccoz, V., Giner Ponce, X y, Vinciperra, R-P. (2006) Las tres estéticas de Lacan, Buenos Aires, Ediciones El Cifrado.
Rodríguez Zoya, L. G. & Aguirre, J. L. (2011) Complexity Theories and Social Sciences. New Nomadic Epistemological and Methodological Strategies, Systems Research and Behavioral Science Syst. Res. 30, 794–796.
Rose, G. J. (1992/1980) The power of form, Nueva York, International Universities Press.
Rosolato, G. (1978) La relación de desconocido, Madrid, Ediciones Petrel.
Serra, P. (2005) "Strangeness, epiphany and late style", El hilo de la fábula. Annual Review of the Center for Comparative Studies (15), p. 33.
Vázquez, M. A. (2007) "Objeto transicional", in "Scilicet: Los objetos a en la experiencia analítica", Buenos Aires, Grama Ediciones.
Winnicott, D. (1971) Realidad y juego, Barcelona, Gedisa.
Winnicott, D. W. (1999/1945) "Primitive emotional development", in Writings on Pediatrics and Psychoanalysis, Barcelona, Paidós, p. 209.
Winnicott, D. D. (1988) Human Nature, London, Free Association Books.

3 The Other in Art and the Dynamics of Estrangement

3.1 Instant experience

The experience of the instant accounts for the notion of time in the aesthetic experience, as estrangement. It is the instant of the encounter with the object of art that, as an event, initiates the estrangement, and generates a temporality inherent to the state of estrangement. It is the temporal correlate of estrangement, and the starting point of that state. Thus, a category is defined that investigates the temporal dimension of the impact of the aesthetic experience that promotes estrangement. It is the instant of the event of the encounter with art, which is in the order of surprise, of something unexpected. That instant is experienced as something unprecedented in the continuity of what is felt, and is separated from other experiences by the unexpected shock it produces in the subject that is, from that moment on, involved as the subject of the experience. It supposes a discontinuity in the chain of time in terms of the dimension of the temporal experience, and a discontinuity, a disruptive impact that crosses the thinkable or expected and moves the body, beyond the word. It is a disruptive, non-traumatogenic event, estrangement as a non-pathological effect. This category of the experience of the instant is characterized as the starting point of estrangement, as the expression of *a privileged instant* that separates itself from the chain of time and acquires a certain consistency, one might say, like the enigmatic phrase from Wagner's Parsifal "*Zum Raum wird hier die Zeit*" ("Here time becomes space"). This shows that, from the shock or surprise of the encounter, the instant becomes the space of estrangement. It is what follows the impact that defines a singular temporality, as outside of time. Therefore, the experience of the instant can be analyzed in two ways: (1) The shock or surprise and (2) time in suspension. Both dimensions are the framework of estrangement; the first is what produces the effect as an instant of the encounter-event that initiates estrangement; and the second is a temporal correlate of the state of estrangement.

The experience of the instant is manifested by irruption: the sudden appearance of an impression caused by art; or rather, by the encounter with the object of art, given that the aesthetic experience has the character of an

DOI: 10.4324/9781003591559-4

"event", an "occurrence", and that, for Adorno, beyond a surprise or shock, is the "happening of a truth", quoted by Jauss. The instant of the event, the instant of the unexpected encounter, is singularly different from other moments and produces a discontinuity in experience and discourse. The instant, in the experience with art "is unique and unrepeatable" as Benjamin states (in Goldstein, 2005). It carries an emotional impact, like a *blow* or a sometimes a soft impact that surpasses logical explanation. That instant is what generates an associative implication that changes the subjective quality in which the sensorial acquires incarnation. It is as if the body felt a particular impact that has nothing to do with the area of the sensory being experienced, which has been captured by the situation, an "entrapment" that corresponds to a sensation of "estrangement". At that moment, words fail. Or else they are insufficient to give an account of the lived experience. It is proposed to be a disruptive effect that implies a shock, an impact, a "being turned upside down" by an encounter with art, which questions us, and makes a truth emerge as something unprecedented. That truth emerges where there is a break in the field of knowledge, since, as Badiou (2000a) states, the event is a break in the field of knowledge of the situation, linked to the unsymbolized truth of the situation. Art is one of the four fields that Badiou delimits as those in which the advent of truth-events takes place (in addition to science, love and politics). In these conditions, art introduces something of that truth, since the encounter with art, as an aesthetic experience, is unexpected, it is an event, which marks a before and an after in the subject's life and reorganizes his psychic economy.

This situation defines the estrangement produced by the event of the encounter with art, a situation that becomes the subject. According Éric Laurent, this state it's like which was described by Lacan as a personal experience in the moments prior to his lecture in Baltimore:

> It was the early morning hours when I prepared this little colloquy for you. I could observe Baltimore through the window and it was a very interesting time as there was not yet full daylight and a neon sign indicated to me every minute the change in the time and there was, of course, heavy traffic, and I emphasized to myself that everything I could see, except the trees in the distance, was the result of thoughts, actively thinking thoughts, where the function that the subjects fulfilled was not entirely obvious. Either way, the so-called Dasein as a definition of the subject was there in this largely intermittent or evanescent spectator. The best image that sums up the unconscious is Baltimore at dawn.
>
> (Laurent, 2003, p. 7)

In this conference in Baltimore, Lacan relates to his audience what we understand as an aesthetic experience, it can be said, in an attempt to account for the emergence of the unconscious, a state of estrangement in which the emergence of the unconscious appears in surprising moments and has the character of an event. Where is the subject, asks Éric Laurent in this article in which he refers to Lacan's anecdote in Baltimore. "It is necessary to propose the subject as a lost object", Laurent asserts. It can be said that in the event that is the experience with art, the subject of experience emerges. The encounter with art is the *encounter with the lost object* in another way, as the possible of that (re)encounter with the object of art that in turn implies something new. In Lacan's terms, it is the encounter with the *real* of the thing, veiled and re-veiled as a lost object; as a condition of desire in that "possible encounter" a function is produced: in agree with Lacan, Recalcati et al. (2006) affirm that the subject find itself as such as "… the function of the painting". Thus, this encounter is a "contingent encounter with what makes the essence of being, the singular feature. A new encounter in the tension between *automaton* and *tyche*, between repetition and chance …", the authors continue. This possible encounter with the real, mediated by the work, implies an auratic, disturbing dimension of the lost object, as a re-edition of something ineffable. "Truth is not at an unreachable distance, but comes to meet us," says Gadamer (1993). He adds: *"The work of art forces us to recognize it. It is an impact, a being turned over, which happens through the particularity with which each artistic experience comes to meet us"* (Gadamer, 1993, p. 91).

Therefore, we understand the estrangement in aesthetic experience as an event, as a non-traumatogenic disruptive event, unlike what happens with the Stendhal syndrome, or the Jerusalem syndrome. The aesthetic experience, as an event, reedits between *tyche* and *automaton*, an ineffable encounter that introduces a truth in the field of something not symbolized, but that, in this "creative disruption" makes the subject of the experience emerge, from the estrangement, in a new creative subjective position, open to the emotions. It summons an effect on the body, a shock for which words fail, and is referred to as impact or sensory immersion, and which refers to the space of the original, as defined by Aulagnier (1997). This experience is lived in an "instant" when time is suspended and dated chronology disappears. This shock from the encounter with art triggers modes of relation between subject and object, between reality and fantasy, between the self and the other, the familiar and the strange, in which there are exchanges that we call creative-poietic from a "poetic disruption". For Benjamin, event and shock are in the category of surprises that, under certain conditions, make that impact "a poetic experience" (in Goldstein, 2005).

The experience of the instant cannot be named and does not remain within associative commerce. The less it is exhausted, the more intense it is, which is why the possibility of exhausting the inclusion in the symbolic will be in the account of the event. This is what Freud says, viewing Michelangelo's *Moses*, when he recognizes that works of art and their overwhelming effects remain obscure to our understanding. He states that one admires them, one feels subjugated by them, but one *cannot say* what they represent (Goldstein, 2005) and goes on to say that something of the "affective situation, the psychic constellation that lent the artist the drive force for his creation" must resonate in us. Nevertheless, he insists on asking: why can't this effect of art *be "grasped" in words* like any other fact of psychic life? These movements that overflow consciousness are enabled by art bridging very subtle modes of drives.

In the category of the experience of the instant, two dimensions can be determined: the first refers to ***shock***, impact or surprise of the unexpected, characterized by a description of an emotional impact for which words are not enough, where the sensory prevails over what can be said, and is of a bodily order. The second is by ***immersion***, where what is described is immersion in an unexpected dimension, which surprises in a different way, like a world or a sea of sensations experienced psychophysically, generally pleasant or dreamlike.

The temporal dimension, time in suspension, alludes to the way time is suspended in the state of estrangement after the impact of the encounter, and is experienced as in a different temporality, where chronological times are superimposed, detached from dated chronology. The first produces the effect as an instant of the encounter-event that initiates estrangement and the second is the temporal correlate of the state of estrangement.

3.1.1 Surprise: Shock, the unexpected

Event and shock, for Benjamin (1973), are in the category of surprises, as an event, and as such, he states, is real experience with "the thing in itself" (*erfahrung*), there "where the insufficient becomes an event" (p. 31), he adds quoting Bergson.

It is the expression of an emotional impact, like a blow to the body that surpasses logical explanation. It can occur in two ways depending on how the instantaneous irruption manifests itself. It can be referred to as such, that is to say, the unexpectedness of something that "appears" "suddenly" or as the "immersion in the sensorial" defined by the intensity of the experience. The instant has the character of shock or surprise, in general, with different degrees of impact, from something experienced with pleasure to psychosomatic impacts: "paralysis", "not being able to move the body", "fainting". Something takes the subject by surprise, because the encounter with the object in the phenomenon of estrangement in aesthetic experience produces an "entrapment" from which not being able to "detach", or "return" are terms that account for this phenomenon. It is as if the body sustained a particular impact in its totality, which has nothing to do with the sensory area being experienced, that is to say, what is *seen*, produces a resonance on the whole corporal plane and, in many cases, promotes an active impulse towards the object such as "touching" or "embracing".

It is the impact evident in the *Spaltung*, or splitting that Freud experiences in Athens, when he was in front of the Acropolis. This is how he describes it in his famous letter to Romain Rolland:

> "When, finally, on the afternoon after our arrival … I stood on the Acropolis and cast my eyes around upon the landscape, a surprising thought suddenly entered my mind: 'So all this really does exist, just as we learnt at school! … a sense of some feeling of the unbelievable and the unreal in the situation at the moment. The situation included myself, the Acropolis and my perception of it" … "These derealizations are remarkable phenomena which are still little understood. They are spoken of as 'sensations', but they are obviously complicated processes, attached to particular mental contents and bound up with decisions made about those contents. They arise very frequently in certain mental diseases, but they are not unknown among normal people, just as hallucinations occasionally occur in the healthy …" "Depersonalization leads us on to the extraordinary condition of' double conscience', which is more correctly described as 'split personality' ("*Persónlichkeitsspaltung*")"
>
> (Freud, 240–241 S E, V22)

The strange "experience" before the Acropolis described by Freud can be understood as the impact of the aesthetic experience that produces a shock, a disruptive effect in the order of the event, which produces estrangement. It is understood as an aesthetic experience, as it is defined. Although for Magherini, Freud may have suffered from a Stendhal Syndrome described by this author, as we said, as a state of disorientation caused by art from Stendhal's story, if we think of it instead from the conceptualizations of modern aesthetics, this experience would be considered a form of aesthetic experience.

In the context of the elaboration of my doctoral thesis, I researched estrangement in the aesthetic experience and its condition as an event. As an example, I include here some fragments of the interviews that show its impact.

In front of Michelangelo's *Pieta* in Rome, one of the interviewees comments on the effect that the surprising sight of the sculpture had on him, and says:

> … *suddenly*, like divine lightning, *La Piedad*, which is placed on a high platform, right? Suddenly it was absolutely illuminated against a black background and against a black backdrop … I remember the feeling that *I was paralyzed* … I stayed with the choir watching, but *without being able to move my body*.

This effect on the body reveals the impact and surprise ("suddenly") and one of the unthinkable reactions, paralysis, as a momentary psychosomatic manifestation. It is a state of temporary estrangement. Another experience refers to another way of describing the physical impact, as "a whiplash in the body", which speaks of the surprise caused by an art installation, in Buenos Aires, in the Recoleta Museum, where there was a black and somber enclosure, with dark masks that were barely noticeable, he says, and points out the most important thing:

> ... it was the rough floor of a very coarse sandpaper ... the rough situation with what was a torture chamber, that was the allusion. What gives you the dimension of torture is the roughness, the helplessness ... It was a feeling of absolute helplessness that would be the opposite of the smooth skin of a woman. This type of experience, which is also a type of experience that appears and disappears, isn't it? This also seems important to me, there are experiences that are *like lightning flashes* that remain engraved, but they have the dimension of *a whiplash*, right?

The factor of surprise and of the impact on the body that is presented as a sensation appears in both descriptions, as well as in the following ones:

> ... In Santa Maria Novella in Florence, which was a very special day because inside Santa Maria I found many things that really moved me because I had a referential relationship with everything I saw or with some of the things I saw. With what I did not have a referential relationship and that *was a surprise,*—there is a square and I go to take a picture—, *I turn around and I see Santa Maria Novella alone as something white*. Is it really white? It is white or is it the idea of *fidanzata (girlfriend)*. It looks painted ....

The experience of the instant, when the impact is referred to as immersion, appears as something unexpected, surprising, although it is not referred to as a blow or shock, the unexpectedness of immersing oneself in a universe of incalculable intensities where the sensitive is described as that which encompasses the experience. The loss of the referential accounts for the event, as defined by Badiou, a break in referential continuity, an event, initiates estrangement.

This immersion in an affective situation is subjugating; it is unexpected and touches a sensitive universe. In these conditions the surprise is that the body seems to float without thoughts and without words, as described by another interviewee, going to the Wailing Wall in Israel and Jerusalem, at sunset and on Shabbat, the Sabbath, when she says:

> ... *suddenly it's as if they lower the audio* and the thing becomes a murmur and it's the light and the colors. It was that instant and the same sensation: no time, no space and being like "oofff", thrown like someone who *throws himself into a pool of sensation*. I had that impression ... I have the same feeling: surprise and something that touches something very intimate ... That feeling of strangeness, of being with me but at

> the same time *floating* and at the same time being there, and for me the intense thing is that there were no ideas … A *state of trance* as such.

The trance, a semi-hypnotic state, like states of sleep or dreaming, are similar to those referred to in amorous experiences, or with art as well, that hint of entrapment.

Shock is about something that cannot be put into words, that touches the *real* of the body, that describes an experience in which surprise is like a plunge into an unexpected and unusual sensitive dimension to which pleasure and complex sensations are summoned. Feelings of nostalgia and loss also account for another form of the experience of what appears in art, which we call the dimension of "the aura", as defined by Benjamin. This experience is a situation that another of the interviewees describes in an exhibition in which there were:

> … huge figures with huge umbrellas and with a kind of relationship of contact between them, a very complex mixture of feelings that conveyed that. That is *a work in which I immersed myself*, isn't it? You saw the kind of contact of the masterfully made bodies and it transmitted an impressive complexity of feelings in that enclosure … It is a fascinating work but there …, the dimension of being on the beach … how they are able to make you feel the helplessness on the one hand and the vicissitude of a life … The transience and the complexity that this transience implies, of course with a *dimension of helplessness* but not the helplessness of violence.

A different, complex and combined sensation is that of the impact that produces paralysis and, at the same time, a sensitive dimension of pleasure and suspension of time and space. What other interviewed describes accounts for the other characteristic of this category. It is an instant in which surprise and shock in the body coincide with the loss of the notion of space and time. It is a situation that determines the experience of the instant of the event and, as described by one of the interviewees under the dome of the Sistine Chapel where she says:

> I was surprised in such a way that you can't stop looking at it …, that is to say, you are speechless … they left me stunned, paralyzed and wanting to stay in that place indefinitely.

In this case, as in other interviews I conducted for the preparation of this research, the dimensions of the phenomenon overlap, giving thickness to the experience, since the impact appears in the "paralysis", while the dimension of the experience of time in the instant is also evident. It is the suspension of time. The allusion to surprise and the unexpected effect, surprise and dumbfoundedness, a state of stupor or unawareness, account for the state of estrangement. This impact is the beginning of estrangement, a state in which these effects: astonishment and "entrapment", are almost inseparable. Entrapment or capture, in that inability to stop looking, in which the drive, and the daze is seduced or hypnotized. The sensation of being paralyzed and speechless is the physical correlate of psychic stunning, the clear manifestation that something of the body is directly touched, in the dimension of the originary, the unconscious drive or, in other words, the *real* as wordless, is at the same time the event, outside the symbolized, even if only for an instant. And then there is an exit from estrangement to pleasure: the desire to stay indefinitely; that is to say, the "desire" already reveals the exit from stupor annihilation. This is an example of how, starting from the instant, the three categories of analysis become intricate, although they are separated in pursuit of understanding of the effect and complexity of estrangement.

3.1.2 Time in suspension, daydreaming

The experience of the instant is characterized by time being *suspended*. It is an ungraspable instant; in the event, it is the moment of encounter with the work. The instant is experience in a "present" time of singular intensity. In the aesthetic experience, it seems that the world is contracted to the work that is being viewed. It seems that we lose the notion of time, and this "instant" that lasts "a thousand years" is separated from chronological time. It manifests itself in suddenness, in being trapped, in returning and returning, with a temporary erasure of the conscious subject absorbed in the scene, as if the subject needed to be called back to the world of everyday reality. Or as Walter Benjamin (1973) puts it: "there must be an emancipation of lived experience (*erlebniz*) in which the present and past are confused undifferentiated. The shock that destroys the usual lived experience puts us in a position to construct a different experience (*erfahrung*) that connects individual memory to collective memory and to history (in Rella, 1981).

In this type of experience, in which there is no opposition between past and present, a new type of memory is promoted, which is not cumulative, but rather lively associative.

In the stories collected, one of the interviewees manifests it when he describes a scene visiting Michelangelo's *Pieta*, in which it seems that time is suspended and the sensation of what is happening is intensified, it is the phenomenon of experience, the privileged instant of the temporality of estrangement.

> ... *it's as if suddenly the world and I were transformed for a second,* wasn't it? It was a kind of wonderful experience, but I must also say that it lasted a little while. *I can't say how long it lasted, possibly in clock time it was just a few seconds, but I do remember the feeling* .... It must have lasted a minute or two minutes because I stayed with the choir watching but unable to move my body ... *I don't remember thinking* anything in particular except the fact of finding myself in front of an extraordinary situation

She seeks to find an explanation for this "loss" of the notion of time in order to understand, but admits that it was something extraordinary. That it involves modes of pleasure, as Juliana also expresses it, in that trip to Israel of which she remembers "something exciting" in the experience of loss of the notion of time as "... something strange ... *I got hung up ... that feeling of strangeness lasted, of being with me, but at the same time floating and at the same time being there. And for me the intense thing is that there were no ideas ...*".

This dimension of experience where time flows can be related to what Agamben affirms in relation to the fact that, in experience, under certain conditions, a liberating dimension emerges when it is articulated "as an inextensive and ungraspable point", with the "idea of pleasure" as the original dimension of man. In these conditions, the question of not being able to express in words or apply reason to account for what is happening and the impossibility of detaching oneself from the experience emerges. In this way it emerges from another story, when being in Amsterdam in the Van Gogh Museum an interviewee comments with astonishment that:

> ... *I was there for five hours; I couldn't take my eyes off the paintings*. It's that thing that transcends that *I can't explain very well in words* ... Especially when I saw the painting of the Yellow Room ... there I went back three times; I walked and went back to the painting, walked and went back to the painting, walked and went back to the painting and at the end I stayed ten minutes looking at the painting. ... *Yes, I totally lost track of time ..., I was surprised to spend almost five hours in the museum, I couldn't believe what I had been there ....*

To lose the notion of time is also to lose oneself in the experience of estrangement in the aesthetic experience, which is also evident in the inability to grasp with words the phenomenon of what is happening to him. Aspects arise in the dimension that, beyond pleasure, *repeat and return* in an experience that exceeds what can be said, so that it can provoke both pleasure and uneasiness.

The entrapment in the experience of the instant refers, already in a state of estrangement, to an "annihilation", a term with which Lacan defines the effect of art, he speaks of an "annihilated" subject, who through the experience with the work, accesses an awakening:

> All this makes us see that in the very realm of the epoch in which the subject is delineated and in which the geometrical optic is sought, Holbein makes visible something that is, quite simply, the subject as annihilated—annihilated in a form that, to tell the truth, is the enlightened embodiment of the less fi of castration ....
>
> (Lacan, 2006, p. 25)

The Eros of form entraps the subject and she loses the notion of time in an extraordinary experience, in which she highlights something in the order of pleasure, beyond annihilation. Another account of her encounter with Michelangelo's sculptures refers to it:

> … it was when *I* met the four men who come out of the stone and don't finish coming out …. That *amazement* has to do with the other sensation of 'I want to stay a while longer to enjoy what I see' …. There is something extraordinary about it … There is an entrapment … I mean, if *at that moment my family had left, I didn't realize it, they had to call me and insist that I leave because I wanted to stay there…, at that moment there were many people but you still abstract yourself from all that where you don't register the noises or the chatter; you are captured by the work in a pleasant way.*

In this story time ceases to pass, for her she is in another reality, estranged, in a state that she refers to as annihilation, (in Lacan terms) but extraordinary. Something of the function of art in the entrapment involved in estrangement compromises forms of pleasure, which the description makes clear. We thus understand that the instant, as we define it, is paradoxical and ungraspable, a pure limit that simultaneously gathers and divides past and future; because, as Agamben states, the instant "is always other"; this is its nature and is the foundation of the radical "otherness" of time. The time of aesthetic experience is also the present… it is an experience that admits, paradoxically, consciousness and the flow of the unconscious in the same time. Time and space merge in a transfigured experience and give shape to what happens in the field of estrangement.

The experience of the instant appears as the expression of the privileged instant separated from time or the loss of the notion of real time. The surprise and unexpectedness of the encounter with art is evidenced as something always different from what was imagined or expected. The dimension of the experience, through the evocative narrative of the interview, recovers affects and resonances with an experience between forgotten and separated in the memory. The impact on the body is highlighted, for which words are not enough, and which in the narrative recovers what is possible of that ineffable and memorable experience, dreamt of and feared in many cases, but in which the sensory dimension leaves room in the narrative for the inference that something of the unconscious, beyond the repressed, was touched in the real. This is how it emerges in several testimonies, where a mixture of paralysis and not being able to detach oneself give an account of the blow to the body, and of the poetic dimension of the event of art. The inference of infinitesimal and complex processes points to the duration of the instant experienced outside of time. These intimate movements, related to tertiary processes, are those referred to by Benjamin: event and shock are, for this author, in the category of surprises, which must remain as an experience with the thing (that resonates in the lost object) since, if memory organizes them, it gives them the time that has been missing, as an event for a poetic experience. Nasio, in turn, speaks of poetic and creative conditions. Thus, the interviews show that the spectator participating in the aesthetic experience who, as Nasio says, creates in turn, lets his unconscious produce something new and unpredictable. "Every human production that includes a part of invention ..., every spontaneous manifestation that surprises the subject and confronts him with himself, is a positive expression of the unconscious that brings something new to the world." (Nasio, 2015, p. 135).

That participating spectator recovers, in the aesthetic experience, portions of experience lost from a sensory dimension that reconnects them with their affections and with new representations, that summon up the story, by means of metaphors and associations and ways of constructing, the ineffable of that touch. The aesthetic experience is event, "shock" and "pacification", a condition of *mediation* that allows, as in creation, access to something new, of the world and of oneself. They are shared experiences, because they belong to the world as cultural goods. The traces of forgotten pleasure, which redraw other traces or coordinates, emerge in the erotic of memory, the *fidanzata* the girlfriend white and perfect, as one of the interviewees said, the skin of the woman in another, the four erotic men of the other interviewee woman, which are manifestations of subjective involvement and mobilization in relation to the affections, the unconscious and erotic desire. Is there a change of meaning or does it make an interweaving in the subjective world? Badiou (2000a), in *Being and the Event* explains that the subject is "*a complex operation*" it presupposes the structure of the situation and a rupture as well. *As if there were a subject only where there is a defect in the structure. This theory of the subject makes it possible to account for phenomena of creation and novelty, and, in this sense, every subject is a novelty* (Badiou, 2000a, p. 6).

It is an encounter that produces a discontinuity of something experienced in an instant whose temporal quality is immeasurable. In that incalculable instant, the intensity of the present sensation, and the influx of the past and the future form a network of unconscious, free associations and sensations. In other words, something of the primordial in the body, the real, the original, enables a potentiality that can articulate a lost experience. The experience to which the aesthetic experience refers accounts for this more or less articulated point between the self and the unknown, identity of perception and identity of thought, the articulation of the internal world with the external world, which is enabled in a state of estrangement.

The experience of the instant shows that it is paradoxical and ungraspable, a pure limit that both gathers and divides past and future; Luis Gusmán (2010) compares it to the "pulsating moment" (p. 51), a privileged moment that Freud granted to the unconscious as an instant in which something of repressed truth is captured before it closes again, which would allow us to think of lucidity ... "as a moment of truth before the opaque resistance of discourse hides it again" (p. 51). Freud enunciates the timelessness of unconscious psychic processes. But at the same time, in the narrative, this experience is included in the symbolic, and wears away or softens its traumatogenic potential. The story in the interviews is the way of referring to something that has happened, since the instant is unique and unrepeatable, and of a quality and intensity different from that of the story. The traumatic experience belongs neither to the order of repression nor to the order of conflict, but is a psychic process of disarticulation generated by not having been able to introject the disruptive impact in an active way. That is to say that, in a sense, the disruptive effect in certain conditions, could preserve its force of poetic experience. The aesthetic experience has included a movement from what appears as "passive" being a spectator, to active, as we propose, as "participant of the experience", that is to say, that participation is one of the characteristics of the aesthetic experience as estrangement and this involves a form of poetic intervention that awakens. In his seminar of 19/04/77, Lacan argues that all discourse has an effect of suggestion that is always numbing, except when it is not understood: then it awakens. The effect of estrangement is closely related, paradoxically, to awakening.

3.1.3 *The moment, event and trauma*

As has already been said, the aesthetic experience is an encounter with the character of an event that involves the subject in an experience with the work of art, that is to say, it involves his participation. It is the object of art, an encounter between subject and object, an encounter that has resonances with the lost object. It is an encounter having specific characteristics. It is a re-encounter with the other, with otherness and with something of oneself, and at the same time, with something strange. It is an effect in the order of surprise, shock or the unexpected, for which words are lacking. It is an encounter with Lacan's real, it is the trauma of the rupture of Freud's anti-stimulus barrier. And it produces a shock in the body. This sudden aspect, as of an irruption, or an instant with super-intense sensory qualities, acquires a certain consistency and separates itself from these experiences. It marks a discontinuity in everyday experience and separates itself sharply.

This encounter with art produces a cut, a discontinuity, in a singular temporal instant, its quality is immeasurable, and the intensity of the present sensation composes the influx of the past and the future as a network of unconscious associations.

In the context of estrangement—the effect of the encounter with the lost object—, associations and lost links are activated and they make consciousness permeable in the flow of a new associative network between sleep and wakefulness, between dream and fantasy. It is the getting lost in the network of associations that promotes the impact, first without words, then with the emergence of unconscious associations. It will be *aprés-coup* in the story where it can be integrated into the discourse by the word or metabolized in a more enriched associative web and in accordance with the subjective work of mourning and loss.

In other words, in estrangement potentiality is enabled that can articulate a sensory, disarticulated experience. It is an effect of creation or creativity given that this encounter, being an event, is discontinuity and production, the potential to create something different or to include the foreign, the other, the raw experience, in an articulated experience, in a transforming and subjectivation potential.

The experience to which the aesthetic experience refers accounts for this more or less articulated point between identity of perception and identity of thought, the articulation of the internal world with the external world.

The notion of *event* within the field of aesthetics is implied in the idea of beauty, argues Gadamer, a scholar of Aesthetics, who finds that it, like aesthetic experience, has the character of an "event", of an "occurrence".

Alain Badiou, in his work *Being and the Event* (2000a) refers to a theory of the subject, where he argues that every subject is something that arises in a structure and at the same time goes through it. However, the subject is not an effect of this structure. The structure as such is a kind of supplement that arises from a chance that he called "event". The event, in fact, is a rupture to this structure, as a phenomenon of creation and novelty, so that every subject becomes novelty, in agreement with what Badiou (2000) and Benyakar (2000) affirm here. In this sense, the aesthetic experience invokes its character of event as a transforming event of the subject.

Benyakar maintains that a disruptive event is "any event or situation with the potential capacity to break into the psyche and produce reactions that alter its integrative and processing capacity" (Benyakar, 2000). This definition tells us about a particular event that can have a direct influence on the subject, involving his psyche. This is where the event arises. Badiou talks about the becoming of the subject, and how it is that, from the moment one is taken beyond oneself in an event, the subject molds and changes, produces and becomes a truth. This transformation, this newness is singular.

However, in addition, the event is a sudden, unforeseeable event that generates a reaction in the subject, although the author would call it a creative chance which, the subject being the source of creation and novelty, he will act as suddenly as the event itself.

From another perspective, it is only in post-revolutionary modern times, with Baudelaire, that other concepts are introduced in the aesthetic experience, such as: the present moment, the shock, and the instant. In "The Work of Art in the Age of Technical Reproducibility" (1973), Benjamin takes up Baudelaire's impressions and incorporates them into a vision that will be representative of a new way of thinking about the aesthetic phenomenon in modern times; it transcends—in its representation by means of contemporary arts (photo, cinema, then installation)—the auratic condition of the work.

The aesthetic experience is an event, a condition of mediation that in turn is an encounter which combines in its consummation the intimate experience of the "felt past with the immediate present," actualizing a type of "sensual" attention, different from that of a drive that seeks discharge. "Time, space and person are re-fused and re-formed, restoring an enriched balance in complexity," asserts Gilbert Rose in *The Power of Aesthetic Form* (1992). This instant of perception, of the immediate present, where the subject produces something previously nonexistent, is in a Deleuzian sense understood as a productive power. "We call productive [...] any power that becomes the cause of what did not exist before," says Deleuze in "An Ontology of the Possible" (1991), a lecture read at the Museo de Arte Contemporáneo Sofía Ímber in Caracas.

It is in that creative process, on that plane of the becoming of the instant-event, according to Deleuze, where representation is in charge of attenuating and filtering the dangerous reality of the random and uncertain presented by the event. In this way, the notion of event is connected to that state of estrangement where a maladjustment is produced in the subject, a de-configuration that allows the emergence of the new.

Following Walter Benjamin (1973) in "The Work of Art in the Epoch ...", that which is perceived "is nothing other than the aura, one whose experience thus lies in the translation of a form of reaction current in human society to the relation of the inanimate or of nature" (p. 21), where, in terms of perception, something is always missing: the here and now of the work of art, always unrepeatable, which promotes the production of something novel. In his developments, Benjamin alludes to a paradoxical sense in relation to the space-time equation of the work of art. The perception of the instant of something enduring and always incomplete that the art object offers. In this sense, Gadamer (1993) argues: "The notion of event in the field of aesthetics is implied in the idea of beauty".

Bolívar Echeverría makes specific reference to the auratic and characterizes the aura "as the halo or nimbus that surrounds the images of Catholic saints", adding that "the Aura of works of art also brings with it a kind of V-Effekt or effect of estrangement [...] that awakens in those who contemplate them when they perceive how in them a metaphysical objectivity overlaps or replaces the merely physical objectivity of the material presence" (Bolívar Echeverria in Benjamin, 1973, p. 27). At the same time, Benjamin argues that the aura is a very special interweaving of space and time: "unique appearance of a remoteness, however close it may be" (p. 27). Thus, the aura refers to an element inherent to the work of art that promotes the viewer's access to a space of interpretation beyond the object and the determined space-time. However, this space of interpretation is also, often and paradoxically outside the discourse.

This quality of being ungraspable by discourse, of incompleteness and evanescence, the appreciation of the instant in which estrangement occurs, all of this can be understood as the mark of the modality of psychic processing set in motion by the subject's encounter with the work of art.

The reference to the ominous as belonging to the field of the originary implies taking up again Piera Aulagnier's developments on the modes of psychic processing. Aulagnier (1997) continues, deepens and broadens certain Freudian problem areas. One of them is her model of the construction and functioning of the psyche, in which she centrally privileges a task: "the activity of representation". In other words, the work assigned to the psychic apparatus involves metabolizing, representing and investing.

Representation is, in these terms, in accordance with what Aulagnier defined as the psychic equivalent of the work of metabolization characteristic of organic activity (1997); that is to say, metabolization is inherent to the activity of representation. It thus assumes a position of continuous, unending metabolization, open to new instances of inscription.

Thus, along with the biological body and the erogenous body, Aulagnier introduces the sensory body; in this register she observes that all sensory functions are also a source of libidinal information. That is to say, the sensory functions recovered from the somatic model inform the psyche in their condition as "sources of excitation and pleasure" or as sources of displeasure or pain. Thus, the perception of the instant, of that event, of the encounter with the art object, in terms of a disruptive event, is coined in sensorial terms, with a clear anchorage in the soma.

It is from here that it is possible to understand the somatic basis of sensations, including the sensation of estrangement (Freudian feeling of estrangement) that will be theorized as a state of estrangement because it refers to the articulation of several components, where the initial shock is its inaugural component which accounts for a moment of disorganization imposed by the aesthetic experience. From there, the plane of emotions (already as relational affects that account for otherness) and feelings (as affects manifested in words within a spatio-temporal continuity) are articulated.

In this line, this encounter with the object of art, in terms of the modern aesthetic experience, transcends the valuation of the sensory as the beautiful and pleasurable; it is what is manifested in the shock of that which moves us as an effect of the "traumatic" necessary in art that resonates in a "version of the spectral" according to H. Foster (2001). This shock alludes, in a circular way, to other qualities of the aesthetic experience, already described, in relation to the encounter with the uncanny or ominous. A quality without which one could not arrive at the aesthetic experience. As Eugenio Trías points out, the beautiful is linked to the sublime and, at the same time, to the mysterious and strange, since without this component at the core of the experience with the object, it does not move. "The uncanny constitutes the condition and limit of the beautiful" (in Goldstein, 2005), he asserts. That is to say, the aesthetic effect cannot occur without being linked to the uncanny present in the work. It is its condition. But it is a condition and a limit: it must be present in the form of absence, it must be veiled, it cannot be unveiled.

Therefore, the aesthetic experience is an event, an encounter and, if it is, it is a middle ground, a paradoxical place of encounter—as I have said—, where the subject is the object of art itself, as a condition of mediation that enables this encounter in the experience.

3.2 Estrangement

As we have been saying, estrangement is the state that enables aesthetic experience. It is the core and condition of possibility of the aesthetic experience, understood as its *neuralgic center*. It is the effect of an encounter with art, with the object of art, with the character of an event that initiates estrangement, as an aesthetic experience. Estrangement is taken in its non-pathological aspect, and outside the definitions of psychiatry. Likewise, in its different meanings, it is understood that in estrangement, there is an action in reference to the subject, and to something that is missed, the lost object, as an inaugural encounter that marks an encounter and a loss, which opens to desire or nostalgia. Some of these issues resonate in estrangement, insofar as the encounter with the art object resonates, in a dreamed reunion, with the lost object, which in turn is underpinned by the condition of the art object, as a polysemic object, which opens to metaphor and evocation: the subject participates and constructs it with his interpretation.

Estrangement as a state refers to a situation, a dimension of estrangement. In this state, object and subject cannot be clearly differentiated, there is an interrelation, a necessary "alienation", outside of pathology. The separation of its qualities is for descriptive purposes and can be organized into the following aspects.

a This "object" of experience is an **ambiguous object** that accounts for intense sensations that alter its perception; sometimes it shines, or the light illuminates it or it has an "undefined form" which also at the same time produce disturbing sensations, since in some way, they question us. This encounter with the "lost object", a specific condition promoted by objects of art and of culture, in their condition as mediation, always refer to something else, as André Green and Elena Oliveras affirm, something either disturbing or nostalgic that refers to something of the lost, and to the desired object in different dimensions: this is the polysemy to which this ambiguity refers, which promotes metaphor and creativity.

b It is characterized by a **sensation of unreality** outside pathology, like being in a dream or part of a story, like an experience of being in scenography, but in the waking state, like an expanded consciousness. It is related to the intermediate area, in Winnicott's words, a zone of illusion, a place that enables "paradoxical thinking" (Zak de Goldstein, 2012). This unreality (sensation) can generate a paradoxical disavowal, i.e. not being able to believe what one sees, or may provoke entry into a metaphorized scene or scene of reverie or fairy tale (it was "like in a fairy tale or a movie") and finally, it grants a condition to the phenomenon linked to a luminous dimension, illumination having a certain proximity to the concept of *insight* (from dazzling to illumination as revelation, or opening that, in turn, is related to the modes of pleasure).

c Finally, **entrapment**, or capture in the experience, what we call "work of art function", a form of "annihilation". It is being captured, "entrapped" and unable to detach oneself from the work, not being able to move in a state of hypnotic trance or paralyzed by the encounter, or as an unintended return towards or around the work, accompanied by complex sensations or various modes of pleasure. It is, in another level of analysis, the movement of the drive, and the "tableau function" that Lacan speaks of in other terms, which brings the subject into being. That is to say, to participate and to construct oneself out of a different place … this involves the subject in the experience with the object. Estrangement as entrapment promotes its participation (or also partition), because in another sense, it "completes" the work by being part of the experience in different ways. It is an encounter between subject and object, in an interplay that is neither conscious nor unconscious. It accounts for an intermediate psychic field or space in the manner of potential space, in Winnicott's terms. It implies in a certain way a momentary subjectivizing alienation in the work, that beyond cathartic or narcissistic identification with the phenomenon or the work, makes the subject emerge from this experience, as the personal examples of Lacan in Baltimore or Freud on the Acropolis, show us. Different dimensions come into play, superimposed, as a polysemic condition of the art object, mediated by predominant ways the subject may appear: a) the oedipal dimension (the forbidden object); b) the auratic dimension, nostalgia for an absolute, transience (the lost object) and c) the ominous dimension, the disturbing, fascinating object (the feared object). The whole aesthetic experience is also the movement of the object and its "altered" encounter, always other. Other and at the same time the cause of desire.

Estrangement (*Entfremdungsgefühl*) or "feeling of alienation", in Freud's terms, a feeling of estrangement that implies living distant from oneself, as an observer of the experience of which one is being a part, points to a phenomenon in which the perception of an object diverges from the rational conviction of this perception. It is associated with alienation as an instant of fusion and indifferentiation between subject and object, in which something foreign, alien to the self or to reality, causes a singular impression and experience. The aesthetic experience promotes estrangement which, in these conditions, accounts for the beginning of the encounter with something other, with the Other as a stranger. It is a border experience, between reality and fantasy, a dimension of experience between dream and wakefulness, between reason and sensation, between the familiar and the strange. Under these conditions "reality" is suspended and the sensory is experienced with great intensity. The sensation of "unreality", compromises modes of pleasure and of something that happens beyond pleasure, which also approaches a "disturbing strangeness", that is, the ominous edge of experience. The variable modes of this strangeness will depend on each person's subjective conditions and singular characteristics. Nevertheless, it is possible to define aspects that characterize this state and the dimension of estrangement. There is a momentary distancing from "objective", effective reality, which appears "altered" in the manner of the dream states of interlude, or as a day-dreaming, a day-dream for Freud. Time is suspended, and an intensified present is experienced as *an extended present*. The sensation is of being there, at that moment, in the midst of an overwhelming, disturbing, pleasurable and strange sensation. Extraordinary. The estrangement in the aesthetic experience is the psychic dimension that enables singular interplay between object and subject. This estrangement shows the risky edge in the instant of experience when perception is permeabilized, as on the threshold of consciousness, which is key to creativity.

The aesthetic experience as an edge experience places us on a threshold, "The doors of perception", as Huxley says (1956), where the differences between reason and sensation are erased, where lived experience (*Erlebniz*), appears in its quality as real experience with "the thing" (*Erfahrung*). It is a (possible) encounter with the Real, as Recalcati affirms, made possible by art, with something immeasurable or ungraspable, also marvelous and strange, for which words are lacking. Between the familiar and the strange, it constitutes a specific form of art and its objects. Thus, we see that estrangement as an aesthetic experience provides a possible strategy, the most appropriate alongside psychoanalysis, to tolerate the strange, the ineffable, the inadmissible of the world and the human condition: "Art represents [is] a strategy against the strangeness of the world", says Jauss (2002).

Estrangement is proposed as the central part of the aesthetic experience, which cannot acquire its profound dimension in terms of the unsettling of the human and the world, and refers to an experience that can be recounted or referred to *a posteriori*. This happens to Freud in the Acropolis, who relates his "strange experience" "a generation later" in a letter to his friend Romain Rolland. Freud refers to something very strange that happened to him in front of the Parthenon in Athens: Freud did not believe in what he saw, to the point of being split into two persons. He says that "this psychic situation of confused appearance", presupposes that "on the Acropolis … I had or could have had this feeling for a time: *'What I see there is not really real'. He defines it: This is called a 'feeling of alienation' (Entfremdungsgefühl)"* (Freud,1936, p. 241). These alienations or estrangements, says Freud, are "like sensations", but it is clear that these are complex processes, knotted to certain contents and connected with decisions about the latter. In the manner of mental mirages in which we want to exclude something from our ego or, in alienations, to disprove a fragment of reality. It is a fragment of reality that appears alien to us (*Fremd*). When the alien is of one's own ego, it refers to a "derealizations"; both alienations and depersonalizations belong intimately to each other", Freud affirms. For Freud, the phenomena of alienation, or estrangement in their universality serve the defense, to keep something away from the ego, to disprove it, and hide its dependence "on the mnemic treasure of the ego and of previous painful experiences that since then could fall under repression …" (Freud 1936, pp. 244–245).

Rosolato (1978), who interprets the feeling of strangeness that Freud describes on the Acropolis as a product of the denial of a reality, that is, of "seeing" what cannot be seen, and affirms that it is closely related to the ominous. Rosolato, likewise, finds that Freud defines in 1910, in a Wednesday record "the feeling of strangeness as the endopsychic perception of the estrangement of the affect, as the libido moves away from one object to another place" (p. 320). Rosolato proposes that the feeling of strangeness (*Entfremdungsgefühl*), unlike the "disturbing strangeness", as the Freudian "ominous" is called in French would allow the subject "to *test* in the aesthetic organization … correspondences and homologies" (Rosolato, 1978, p. 339) that, by making them vary through the "game of disavowal and metaphor-metonymic oscillation, allow the subject to abandon himself to the strange, to surprise as unknown" (p. 339) because it consists in *experiencing* "the object's contradictory structure". This specificity of estrangement in the "aesthetic organization" of which the author speaks, coincides with the notion proposed as estrangement in the aesthetic experience, in that abandoning oneself to the strange, which promotes creative potentialities by enabling the object's "contradictory" structure as something that opens to metaphor and metonymy. Under these conditions, a non-pathological disavowal and *dialectical splitting* are possible aspects of the creative processes of estrangement (Goldstein, 2005).

The alienating moment, or estrangement, is the central point of the aesthetic experience, in which a truth-nucleus emerges, the truth of the unconscious, as the Other and the self, as what is missing in what is lost, the subject as a lost object. In the state of estrangement, it emerges as a revelation that the self is not unique and coherent, since by admitting the split, it admits that the self is also other (*car je est un autre*, in Rimbaud's words). The other becomes self and the self becomes alienated in the other, showing the dialectical function of alienation and separation of self/non-self that construct subjectivity from the times of identification jubilation. It is related to the instant of recognition that accounts for the feeling of being alive and of "Here I am!", the experience of being alive, lived subjectively, which Lacan, in the Mirror Stage defines with the interjection of enthusiasm: *Aha* (*Erlebnis*). In the same line, Winnicott gives an account of the I and the not-I in the space of culture, constituted from the potential intermediate space, when he affirms: "The place of cultural experience is the potential space that exists between the individual and the environment, the times of the first experiences that exist between the subjective object and the object perceived in objective form, between the extensions of the *I and the not-I*" (Winnicott, 1971).

I coined the term "dialectical splitting" (Goldstein, 2005) in the aesthetic experience to denote the admission of doubt sustained in non-pathological aspects of estrangement: we take upon ourselves the possibility of experience that admits the irruption of the unconscious and the "strange" aspects of the self and of the world, in a dimension that opens to forms of creative processing.

From another point of view, art offers an aspect that Adorno understands as "apparitions", since this aspect "implies the irruption into reality of something unforeseen and unthought-of, comparable to an explosion" (Perniola, 2001, p. 140), according to Perniola (2001, p. 140);. he goes on to say that "the adequate notion to grasp the essence of art from the cognitive point of view is for Adorno (2004) that of "enigma" (p. 113), since this author (Adorno) affirms that works of art necessarily put us in relation "... with that strange and heterogeneous dimension with which every true work of art is continually confronted". Then, citing Merleau Ponty's point of view, he says that the "artistic emotion par excellence is the sense of estrangement with respect to empirical life, accompanied by a kind of amazement at the existence that is reborn in every experience" (Adorno, 2004, p. 142).

We propose that outside pathology and in intimate relation with aesthetics, estrangement is an essential characteristic of the aesthetic experience, since in that "state" or "sensation", the condition of the possibility of such experience, the encounter between subject and object, is realized, although in a different state: "unexpected" or, we could say, extraordinary.

In this sense, we see that, for Adorno, "the act of estrangement in that objectification that every work of art carries out is corrective" since "in every genuine work of art something appears that does not exist" (2004, p. 113). Estrangement is a psychic "movement", a condition of the aesthetic experience: the impact of the encounter as an event, initiates and promotes this distancing from empirical reality: in one case, it produces a radical disavowal and the ominous appears in another case, the distancing produces the effect of graduating proximity from the object and being able to "contemplate" it, resting the gaze on it and allowing oneself to be carried away by sensations, affects and associations. This losing oneself in estrangement initiates an uncalculated unfolding of affects and associations following the instant of impact that, in estrangement, challenges the subject in that dimension of the genuine work of art that makes something that does not exist "appear". In this subtle psychic movement, the affectivity summoned may reach painful or nostalgic or erotic memories, but muffled by art, enabling a new field of experience in subjectivity. In clinical work, by activating what is disarticulated, heterogeneous and potentially traumatogenic in a measure enabled by art, it offers the possibility of articulating the experience with a new trace, creatively.

Estrangement as an effect of the encounter with art, being a passage zone, gives rise to the *space of experience* that, as an *alienating threshold,* enables the phenomenon of aesthetic experience. Therefore, it is a central characteristic of that experience and the effect of the encounter in that *mit* "with", the "middle point" in the aesthetic experience. It is a phenomenon promoted by the encounter with art, with a work of art, with the object of experience. That object, as mediation, is the "lost object", which in these conditions "brings forth the subject". This is what Lacan recognized when he said in Baltimore in 1966: "It is necessary to find the subject as a *Lost Object*. More precisely this Lost Object is the support of the subject" (in Laurent, 2003). It is the "ineffable encounter" that touches the originary, an encounter with the *real*, following Lacan, that promotes estrangement and a particular form of pleasure. It is, in other words, the encounter with the strange, with the Other, in its radical otherness and in the ineffable quality of the experience. It is a form of *creative involvement* in *being part* of the experience, rather than being just a passive spectator. But at the same time, "touching that" and being moved, produces some kind of pleasure, which implies a form of "awakening" as an event, or unexpected effect: *something else* also happens and, the strangeness of the experience, is what introduces the aesthetic experience.

In Freud's account on the Acropolis, we find the different aspects of estrangement: denying reality by not being able to believe what he sees is part of a form of paradoxical denial. The sensation of such unreality leads him to figure a monster in what he sees, and the separation into two persons accounts for the impact of the shock of the instant and the commotion in the *real* of his body: the unconscious was touched and appears, appears to him in act. Then, the way he reacts to the encounter with "something so desired", which appears as an ambiguous object, shows the estrangement and some of its characteristics.

The sensation of estrangement as something marvelous, which Freud relates to a specific sensory quality of screen memories and *Fausse reconnaissance*, is included in the category of the marvelous and ominous. Freud calls "sensation" "that which moves us in all these moments; it is undoubtedly a judgment and indeed a judgment of discernment" (Freud, 1901, p. 257). That is to say, it shows that something escapes comprehension and the possibility of discerning reality. In estrangement, it is a necessary condition for the effect of the encounter with art to promote a dimension of aesthetic experience.

In the interviews carried out during research, with one of the interviewees, the effect of estrangement reaches an extreme point, almost Stendhalian, which she can formulate as "… a moment where you say 'Where am I?'", of the order of "… *a very brief depersonalization*" that is disturbing and almost ominous, in which "… one wants to be in oneself again, one does not want to live in that sensation", which happens to her when visiting the ruins of Pompeii, which she describes:

> … at one point we were touring Pompeii … and I had a very strange physical sensation of discomfort. Everything made me feel short of breath or that I didn't like being there … at one point I see a group of

> people going to a window and I move away from my acquaintances and go to that window. When I look through the glass, I see a family with children as if alive in their positions, they were dead, with the effect of the lava. I approached the glass to get a good look because I could not believe what I was seeing and I thought I was falling to the ground and luckily, I was saved.

In this case, we see how the intensity of the experience as estrangement approached the ominous without mediation, whereby the phenomenon reached a threshold—at a point of maximum commotion—that reached something in the order of the disruptive in the estrangement in the experience.

3.2.1 Ambiguous object

The object of aesthetic experience becomes an object of doubt, reflecting a specific characteristic of art objects, which can be one thing or another; it is the plurivocity that corresponds to the art object in its *metaphorizing potential*, it is something and it is not; it appears with a difference between the object of perception and the object found, which is never exactly the same as what was expected or imagined; it maintains a difference that is specific to it in its condition of paradoxical object, or appears as "something" that cannot be clearly identified; its paradoxical condition is characteristic of the object of estrangement that art objects promote as an aesthetic experience. This is what becomes evident in Freud's experience, when the Acropolis becomes an object of doubt, something ambiguous somewhere between marvelous and ominous. It is what *La Pietá* becomes when one of the interviewees describes the strange thing that happens to him when he visits St. Peter's:

> I am in the first nave of St. Peter's and this happens on the far right and I enter from the far left, so I have the whole width of St. Peter's in front of me. Seen this way, it was very important because it did not allow me to see what was happening and then it is as if suddenly … I find this *white object, which I know what it is, but I find it floating in the air in a black frame illuminated* with music and I, I do not know how long the nave of San Pedro is, between 60 or 70 meters, with which that very strange feeling of seeing it floating in the air more or less because it was very dark, the people were dressed in dark [clothing] and it gave the feeling of something strange.

That "something strange" that he suddenly finds turns out to be an ambiguous object "… I find this white object, which I know what it is, but I find it floating in the air …".

This object, floating in the air, "something strange", turns out to be an ambiguous object. This "I find this white object, which I know what it is, but I find it floating in the air" seems to refer to what Recalcati says in relation to the work of art and aesthetics when he affirms that "there is a work when there is an encounter with the stain, with that which pierces the purely representative framework of the semantic organization of the work" (Recalcati et al., 2006, p. 24).

It is the characteristic ambiguity of the object of aesthetic experience as defined by Paul Valéry, in *Eupalinos or the Architect* when he describes a dialogue between Socrates and Phaedrus, who, walking along the edge of the sea, encounter *L'objet du monde le plus ambigu* ("the most ambiguous object in the world"), something irrupts, "one of those things that the sea throws up; *a white thing, of the purest whiteness; polished, hard and light* ...", he says. What was the strange object that Socrates throws into the sea? Jauss points out that, in that instant, "he becomes a philosopher," as Elena Oliveras (2005) recalls.

It is the ambiguity the object recovers, the multivocity of its significance and its evocative power, which appears in a similar way in what another of the participants of my research describes, when in Florence he visited the Church of Santa Maria Novella, and comments:

> ... in Santa Maria Novella in Florence ... it was when I was coming out with my head pounding from seeing so many works ... and I turn around and I see Santa Maria Novella alone as *something white*. I remember that I was impressed ... *suddenly I see Santa Maria Novella all in that pure front. I remember that it was a thing of time and purity but not of ruin, not that purity of the past but that active purity, no? and sensual. There was present that idea of my fidanzata.*

And referring to Michelangelo's name for her, "*fidanzata*" he goes on to say:

> She is charming, she is prefect ... she is my *fidanzata*. I remembered that phrase of Michelangelo and it was exciting because you understand it; it is a love for a young girlfriend from when one is young too. "My girlfriend" but the word in Italian is much more because it has a promise. There was no one there because I went in winter, there was no one there and there were no tourists. That image of Santa Maria Novella; *white. is it really white*?

The interviewee is surprised by "something white" that makes him doubt, and he speaks of purity and associates it with the purity of a bride, "my bride", and continues doubting, before the facade of the church that as an object of ambiguity leads him to other associations and metaphors, which involve him in the full power of estrangement in the aesthetic experience, where the ambiguous object takes him back to ideas and sensations of the order of sensuality and the ideal, "alone as something white" ... that front so pure. ... That image of Santa Maria Novella, white. "Is it really white?" he wonders.

Does it have white or is it the idea of *fidanzata*? "It looks painted ...", he says. The ambiguity of the object, which transforms and appears as something else, leading him from sensation to erotic and nostalgic ideas and feelings. "The ideal bride." Something of the amorphous, appears, which Recalcati, calls "anamorphic aesthetics" (as the second aesthetics in Lacan), which aims to make possible the encounter with the real whose object, he says, appears "suspended" and "oblique" and is what operates "an ominous rupture of the familiar" (2006, p. 17). This is what Lacan illuminates from Holbein's painting *The Ambassadors*. In this painting a white stain, oblique, ambiguous appears, which can only reveal the enigma in the "cipher" of transience, when looked at from a slant. This makes "possible" an "encounter with the real", something that escapes symbolization. This aesthetics are constituted "on the constituent ambivalence of the Freudian ominous", according to Recalcati. This ambivalence is revealed in another of the experiences collected in my study, when it is not possible to explain what happens to an interviewee in front of a sculpture, which is an ambiguous object, when she relates:

> ...Once we went to the Picasso Museum in Paris and I remember there was a *very simple stone* carving *and I stayed for about half an hour and I don't know what I was looking at because it was extremely simple and flat*. I don't know what fascination I had, I asked myself "What am I doing looking at this for so long?.

Here we see the disturbing effect of fascination; the ambiguous object of Valéry ("extremely simple and flat stone") whose effect disconcerts her and at the same time interrogates her. That it questions us is another characteristic of art objects, because great works question us and make us "philosophize"; that is to say, beyond aesthetic pleasure, in its ambiguous condition, it promotes a form of thought in non-thinking, as Rancière proposes in the aesthetic unconscious. The object that in estrangement is literally experience of the edge, in the case of Susana. She refers to her experience at the Twin Towers Memorial of their fall on September 11, 2011 and describes what she experienced at the disturbing depth of a hole and what is not seen, the emptiness that lies beyond the visible and the decipherable. I find the object, as a "hole", a void, around which there are "names", words, to sustain the unsustainable, the impact of "pure trauma", the crash and fall of the towers, configured in a work. This object accounts for what Recalcati says, following Lacan, insofar as "art as organization of the void" puts in relation the real of the thing, that is, the bordering of the void, understood as that which organizes and circumscribes, the thing as the limit of the representation of "vortex" or "abyss that aspires" (Recalcati et al, 2006, p. 13), beyond the unrepresentable, which is described in another account:

> … The last thing I found moving is the monument they have made where the Twin Towers fell, it's something else. Right at the base square of each Tower, they have made a fountain with walls around it where *the water falls inwards to a bottom that you can't see. All around are engraved in bronze the names of the victims*, grouped by zone or group to which they belong; those on the plane, the firemen, the employees, etc. I thought nothing was going to happen to me, it moved us all equally, it shook all four of us.

And she continues:

> I can't explain it, I don't know what the conception or the idea of that moment was, but the truth is that it moves you and gives you an idea. *The water falling to the bottom that you don't see gives you a dimension of what happened that goes beyond what you read in the newspapers or the tower you see falling on television, it goes much further ….*

This dimension of estrangement captures the profound dimension of the experience that touches the subject and moves him in the body. This "possible encounter" with the real has a meta-psychological correlate with the lost object, the object and its trace, the resonances of the thing, "*das Ding*", the thing, which recovers the power of its multivocity, in the emptiness, the hole left by it. And which, at another level of analysis, is related to the mother, forbidden and incandescent object. The encounter with art accounts for a "signifying bordering around … of the thing …" in which "Lacan notices the double status of the Thing in a work of art (lost object… but also condition of existence of the signifying chain) in a work of art …" (Recalcati et al. 2006, p. 17).

The statute as "double of the thing" can be associated to the idea of ambiguity of the object, as a condition of the object of art and psychoanalysis.

Likewise, from another point of view, Green describes the object from different dimensions and puts it in relation to Lacan's (*a*). We agree with the idea of the object as *mediation* "the element of the indispensable mediation that unites the subject with the Other", says Green in *Metapsychology Revisited* (1995). Later he adds: "In the range of its variants, between the lack and the imaginary, we propose an indirect or ambiguous tide, as an indispensable 'third term' for the structuring of the subject" (Green, 1995, p. 195). This mediation, third term, accounts for an object "in relation" as it is proposed in the dimension of estrangement in the aesthetic experience, in which tertiary, potentially creative processes occur imperceptibly. In this way, what we propose as potentiality arises from the question of what comes before the loss of the object, that is to say "if it is not appropriate to link together, by the traces, this loss with the attempt to erase these traces", which relaunches the (*a*) as "the path of a hand that traces, inscription, letter, *a*" (Green, 1995, p. 201), writing and gesture related to the creative processes, as tertiary processes.

Ambiguity in psychoanalysis, thought of as a potentially creative vector, has in turn intersections with what Meltzer describes in *The Apprehension of beauty*. It is the ambiguity that occurs in the encounter with the mother's face and her enigmatic interior that activates the aesthetic conflict and the apprehension of beauty.

In estrangement as an aesthetic experience, there is a movement between the impact of the encounter with the ambiguous object and a form of distancing that produces, at the same time, a pacification of the gaze and an "awakening". It is the encounter with the thing, "in German *das Ding*" to which Freud refers in the "Project..." (1895) in relation to the lost object, which appears, in turn, as alien. In the complex of resemblance, Freud relates it in turn to a perceptual complex of characters united as an unassimilable thing. "It is the lost object as such. And Lacan points out in Seminar 10:

> "...that object, as the absolute Other of the subject, is what one tries to find again, one only finds it again as longing, one does not find it again, the only thing one finds again are its coordinates of pleasure".

3.2.2 *Feeling of unreality-Zone of illusion*

This dimension of estrangement refers to the experience described by the subject, understood as his psychic state in the lived experience of estrangement. It is the particular description of the state in which he/she finds him/herself. It is a sensation of unreality, outside of pathology, in which reality is transformed and seems like a dream or a story in which one is taking part. The experience of estrangement is lived as an immersion in something pleasant or very disturbing. The essence of the sensation of estrangement is that of something incredible or unreal, as described by Freud in his experience on the Acropolis when he says that "the original must have been a feeling that in the situation at that time *something incredible and unreal* was registering". *It was a situation that included his person, the Acropolis, and the perception of Freud himself*, who says that "this psychic situation of confused appearance" implies that [about the Acropolis] "I had or could have had for a time this feeling: '*What I see there is not in fact real*'. This *is called* a 'feeling of alienation' (*Entfremdungsgefühl)*". "They are described, Freud states, "as "sensations", but it is clear that these are complex processes, knotted to certain contents and connected with decisions about the latter... in the manner of the occasional hallucinations of healthy people... like dreams... their regular occurrence in the healthy." This is the core of estrangement: unreality, disbelief, disproof, hallucinations or something like in dreams. And all this is defined, according to Freud, by estrangement, in which sensations are the way they are described. In this context Freud understands that it is about what cannot be seen, or is not believed possible, other than by accounts or through study, as when he refers to his disbelief before the Acropolis ("Then all this actually exists just as we learned it at school!"). It ranges from the doubt of the existence of what is being experienced to the alteration of what is seen, or the encounter with a different reality.

This other reality in relation to the encounter with art is referred to by Gilbert Rose as a "fluid reality" when he states that there is "a dialectic between control and ambiguity", assimilable to an oscillation between primary and secondary that gives rise to an interplay between tension and discharge (Rose, 1992, p. 46). It is about the way in which it configures a space between subject and object in which it occurs, in a kind of sensitive and thinkable dimension, as if it were a dream, but being awake, where fantasies or reveries are part of that instant; it is characterized by the intensity of what is perceived that is referred to as sensation. The sensation of being part of a movie, a story, or something referred to as narrated or seen in a book, acquires reality, and this has a surprising effect on diverse modes of pleasure. Metapsychologically, the dynamic is one *between* primary and secondary processes, as in an oscillating coming and going, which creates a space of experience in which other kinds of processing, called tertiary, take place, and a form of psychic occurrence that admits pleasure and the reality principle, sensation and thought, at the same time. Tertiary processes, following Green in *Metapsychology Revisited* (1995), put primary and secondary processes in relation: "… together with primary and secondary processes, it was necessary to create a third type of processes that I call tertiary" (p. 186). He defines them as processes that put the two in relation, avoiding saturation at either extreme. He adds: "This relationship constitutes an unstable equilibrium associated with the constitution of a field of illusion described by Winnicott. In it, states Green in *Metapsychology Revisited* (1995) says: "the work of thought […] consecrated to the exercise of secondary processes, remains open to primary processes that ensure the irruption of creative intuition at the very moment of exercising the most rigorous rationality" (p. 186).

Tertiary processes are the source of creative processes, as Zukerfeld (2002) and Fiorini (2006) argue. It is then about what happens in that *in-between*, that is to say the dynamics in the intermediate or potential area, Winnicott's intermediate zone. It is the cliché of the space of estrangement as an aesthetic experience, in which its edges may border on the ominous that produces the blurring of the boundaries between the real world and a "fantastic created world". That is to say, it is between primary process and secondary process, between effective reality and fantasy, between external world and internal world where we propose that the complex dimension of this experience unfolds. This is the dynamic at play in estrangement, between subject and object, in the situation of experience. The topic is that of the instant transformed into openness to what happens in this complex potential space, a poetic zone of illusion and estrangement. "If only we could discover in ourselves or in our peers an activity somehow akin to poeticizing!" says Freud in "The Creative Writer and the Day-dreaming" (1908). We take up his inquiry in the hope of obtaining a first clarification about creating. He finds in the child the first traces of the poetic task, when "he inserts the things of his world in a new order that pleases him [...] he employs in its great amounts of affect" and he clarifies: the opposite of playing is not seriousness, but ... effective reality. "Now, from the unreality of the poetic world derive very important consequences for artistic technique...", Freud continues in the aforementioned article. It is the place of reverie. From another point of view, it is an intermediate place, Winnicott's potential space, which defines a "zone of illusion". We understand that, in this zone or space, psychic states are produced which, as estrangement in the aesthetic experience, are specific to it and are part of the phenomenon that makes up its characteristics. Three subcategories are proposed: from the non-pathological denial of reality or perception to the sensation of being in a story or a dream, but awake. The luminous dimension is an emergent of the interviews that surfaced as an essential element, since it has the character of "illuminating a scene", as in theater and scenography, of dazzling, or as when one doubts the object that seems to shine, as an apparition that may be blinding. The illumination is like accessing a dimension of semi-dreaming, intermediate states of sleep where the scene that is viewed produces pleasure and experiential effect and contributes to create the scene in which the lighting gives depth and warmth. It refers in turn to different modes of pleasure.

3.2.2.1 Paradoxical denial

That which is seen is considered unreal (the highest degree of distortion of reality or perception, "what I see is not real", says Freud). He is astonished that something desired is considered unreal: this is in relation to what is thought to be impossible, when it becomes reality and to a certain singular condition in relation to desire, as Freud formulates it on the Acropolis. However, Mannoni (1973) relates the idea of mechanisms that sustain a reality while at the same time disproving it, not necessarily pathological, or in other structuring senses. These mechanisms are in relation to belief and operate beyond repression. "I know, but yet", Mannoni states, as from Freud's *Verleugnung* Lacan's imaginary, accounts, according to Mannoni, *"that there is no unconscious belief and belief presupposes the support of the other"* (Mannoni, 1973, p. 8). What cannot be seen, but was known, seen or studied, which appears to be unbelievable or different or unexpected, enters the dimension of the split, beyond repression and outside pathology. This dimension manifests itself from the radical doubt regarding what is being seen to the alteration of what is being seen or the encounter with a different reality. This is what an interviewee describes when, viewing a painting by Van Gogh, he refers:

> "In front of Van Gogh's little painting, you know what I felt: "this painting is a lie and this painting is not the real one"; in the painting it seems that the window and the chair pop out and I said "it can't be! This painting is a reproduction... in other words, a disbelief in one of these works... "here, they lied to me"

In this case, the denial of the work, something the interviewee explains does not always happen to him, or at least, with music it does not happen to him, gives an account that he cannot believe in *what he sees*. This also happens to Freud on the Acropolis when he exclaims, *"Then all this does indeed exist just as we learned it at school!"*, a doubt that reaches denial, and the *Spaltung* outside pathology, which highlights the character of estrangement, when he associates the incredible with the vision of something unbelievable and ominous. "With slight exaggeration: it is as if someone, strolling in Scotland along Loch Ness, suddenly saw the body of the much-talked-about monster slithering ashore and was forced to admit: "So there is indeed this snake in the loch that I did not believe in!", says Freud in his letter to Rolland. It is (following Freud) the momentary admission of a fragment of truth introduced into consciousness, unexpectedly, as something very strange that we want to disprove. "What I see there is not in fact real", Freud declares before the Acropolis. Manonni (1973) affirms that by virtue of having lost that "other scene" the fantastic is nothing other than fantasy, that is, it recovers something of the fantasy rejected in "the world in which we live".

But why such disbelief in regard to something that, on the contrary, promises high pleasure, Freud asks himself before the Acropolis, "A truly paradoxical behavior!". Freud mentions a delayed effect *{Nachwirkung}* on the Acropolis; "I was then forty-eight years old," he says. "According to the testimony of my senses, I am now standing on the Acropolis; nevertheless, I cannot believe it," he writes. "Well then, in this disbelief, this doubt in a fragment of reality…", he expresses. He reminds the king that he does not want to accept his defeat, the fall of the Alhambra, he does not want to "consider it true" {"wahr *haben*"}. And Freud says: "Such a disbelief is obviously an attempt to disavow a fragment of objective reality, but there is *something strange* in it," he says, and astonished he denies, at the same time as he sees. This extreme effect in estrangement refers to a mode of psychic functioning, disavowal and splitting, but outside of pathology, which in estrangement open a field in which modes of psychic functioning, can later become metabolizations, are the supreme effects of art that, in estrangement, give rise to passions and drives. In this sense, Nasio (1994) speaks of two major effects on the spectator of works of art: they hypnotize him and simultaneously arouse the same creative passion that led the creator to produce his work." "That hypnosis in art awakens our creative impulses" (Nasio, 1994, p. 112–113). In a way, this is what happens to the participant, a music teacher, as an impulse that accounts for the intensity of the estrangement effect, when he tells what happened to him in relation to a painting by Vermeer, and says:

> "It also happened to me… I touched a painting… I touched it. I was alone in Amsterdam, Holland, in front of a Vermeer and I said 'I touch it', it was a feeling of having it and 'I have it here. I have this painting here". Two doors open and a tall, big, black man appears and asks me

> "Are you all right?" I say "Yes, I'm very well". "Do you know what you did?", "Yes", "You know it is totally forbidden."

This interviewee shows a high level of estrangement, in which there is a denial of perception that drives him to an action. He does not just think that he could not believe what he saw. The denial of reality drives him to "touch" the painting, even though he knows that it is forbidden and can have consequences, such as what happens next. The aspect of the disavowal and the irresistible impulse not only shows the childish aspect elicited as access to the forbidden, but also the estrangement he experiences, which makes him disavow reality, what he sees and the prohibition. This happens in the aesthetic experience as estrangement that causes the subject to be captured by the experience, in a capture zone, and allow himself to be fascinated by the work, as Nasio says. In the case of this participant, it translates into an impulse to touch, as a "creative" impulse, that is to say, one's own, and transgressive as "creation" and a "touching". The eye touches what it looks at, as Freud says in "Three Essays…", but the dikes inhibit the action. In this state of estrangement, however, it goes beyond what is looked at, imposing an action or what, in another context, would be a passage to the act. The aesthetic experience as estrangement implies a form of capture and of allowing oneself to be captured, since the place of estrangement is the place of capture, which enables a zone, as if hypnotic, where the direct creative aspects of the drive appear.

3.2.2.2 A scenery, a tale, a dream

This dimension is characterized by being experienced as the middlst of a scene, a dream or a story, in which the interviewee is the protagonist. Reality acquires the consistency of a dream, a play, or a scenography, where figure and background are clearcut in the manner of a scene, but in wakefulness. These situations are described in a state of estrangement. Situations *reanimated by an impression* that the effects of art evoke through its effects in the estrangement, which the light or a glimpse transforms the experience into a stage, as happens in the theater. In estrangement, the effect of art evokes a blurring of the boundaries between the real world and a fantastic, created world. It makes a strange appearance irrupt surprisingly, showing something that escapes the conscious. The blurring of boundaries between reality and fantasy, between thought and perception, are a central part of estrangement in the aesthetic experience as unreality.

In this dimension where the sensory is a priority, the dream-like experience has the intensity that Freud gives to screen memories, which are characterized by a sensory intensity that makes them "ultraclear," and are constructed, according to Freud, "like a literary creation, so to speak," and he continues: "It seems, moreover, that in and of itself the memory of a remote past is facilitated by a motive of pleasure. *"Forsan et haec olim meminisse iuvabit"*. (Perhaps, one day, even this will be enlivened by memory [Virgil, Aeneid, I, 203] in Freud, 1899, p. 310) and says that these "mnemic remains of childhood, the screen memories treated here, can be treated as heterogeneous elements [...] And in this precise case, given the thick sensory intensity..."; he relates them to childhood memories, whose "entirely plastic configuration, only comparable to those represented in the theater".

Analogously, in dreamwork and its concern for figurability, images are designed, joining energy from one trace to another, by condensation and displacement in transferring movement in which time is the present. Dreams also make use of the present. The representational movement in the dream is regressive in its hallucinatory animation of images and perceptual traces; if this current started from the unconscious and continued in wakefulness, this process would be "progredient". We propose that "in the aesthetic experience, in a tilting movement, the progredient and the regressive sense" are superimposed in a dynamic from which other forms of psychic functioning result (Goldstein, 2005). In this dynamic of coming and going, between primary and secondary process that is enabled in the state of estrangement, the so-called tertiary processes become manifest. This temporal simultaneity in the aesthetic experience of which we are a part, is "an experience that admits, paradoxically, the conscious and the flow of the unconscious at the same time. How does this superimposition happen? Time and space merge in a transfigured experience and give shape to that which happens in a field inherent to the event" (Goldstein, 2005). It is there that the very movement of transposition appears, represented by images as a visual manifestation of the libidinal charge of the object. This representational production exposes the effect of transference from past to present, from percept to image, and is an expression of the nexus of that which circulates in a "between" space. It is the work of bonding itself that gives form to what is inherent to the aesthetic experience. In the aesthetic experience there is a thirdness in the dialectic between the subject of the experience and the inexorable object of art, a symbolized object of culture, enabled in the state of estrangement, that leads us to a new elaboration of the primary and secondary processes in interrelation: these are tertiary processes that involve a more highly elaborated production, in the sense of sublimated drive. In the estrangement of the aesthetic experience, dreams and daydreams, it underpins its objects, objects of desire in a created object that, expropriated from subjectivity, is an object of culture; this is already a condition that it symbolizes by introducing the tertiary factor. This is how another of the participants in the study describes her experience at the Wailing Wall in Jerusalem when she recounts immersing herself in that state, between sleep and wakefulness, as a threshold of perception where sensations are intensified, experiencing herself as part of a scene or a film. In the manner of the Freudian screen memories, the olfactory (as in Proust) and the sensory mark the pattern of this psychic state, as in dreams or fantasy, but awake. Losing oneself in this reverie is pleasurable, as she describes it:

> "…At the Wailing Wall it was more like it takes over your whole body, now I remember sometimes I've thought whether this was also inaugural, isn't it… in Kurosawa's films where things come to life, some of that unexpected too…".

And she continues:

> … Now that Kurosawa film *Dreams* comes to mind, where he gets into Van Gogh's painting and I think there is something of that, like you get into that work and a time/space parenthesis opens up, which is that of the experience that is an instant ….

And she repeats that "it was something exciting … it was something strange … I got hung up" (it would be the expression of being carried away by an intermediate state). The dimensions of the theater, ("as if they had opened a curtain"), scenography, the scenographic lighting, and "entering a painting" refer to this scenographic dimension of estrangement, a screen of representation is broken, fiction becomes real but, in this case, a pleasurable unreality. Unforgettable.

Similarly, another interviewee describes a situation and a state in which the notion of reality and dream merge in an experience where something strange and unreal appears as if entering a scene, also as marvelous, of a mystical nature, and refers:

> We psychiatrists call it that feeling of "depersonalization and 'derealization' but not with anguish, but *as if suddenly the world and I had been transformed for a second, right? Let it be clear that it is not with an unpleasant sensation, on the contrary, it was a kind of wonderful experience …*".

That experience of intensity where the real and concrete world where she lives - as one of the participants narrates it - as estrangement, "… as if suddenly you were not happening or I was not in that real and concrete world; but as if suddenly a sort of scene had been set up …" *and being part of a scene* occurs, in his case, in an exemplary way considering the characteristics of the description of her experience, as well as the qualities of the sensations, which reach a sort of "depersonalization" and being part of a scene is given, in her case, in an exemplary way in the characteristics of the description of her experience, in terms of the qualities of the sensations, which reach a kind of "depersonalization and derealization" in her words, as Freud refers to it on the Acropolis in relation to estrangement. In other cases, this living in a story or scene appears in the reference to a lived scene, in which the subject suddenly does not know if it is a dream or a fantasy, because at that moment of estrangement, the imagined or dreamed and the incredible of seeing or believing are amalgamated in the experience, with the encounter with art or culture, in another of the stories:

> … something foreign … Because you always see it from the outside and then because those places have a history that adds a magic to them. *You imagine yourself inside the movie, for example the Woody Allen movie that came out of the screen, it's something like that. You are in Venice and they tell you that "prisoners used to pass by on that bridge" and you say "this is me". You are immersed in a story or a fable.*

In this case, the scenographic quality is organized as a situation where the difference between reality and story or fantasy is blurred or permeabilized, in a type of experience like seeing oneself in a story or in a movie and at the same time having lived the experience. When she says "… *You imagine yourself inside the movie, for example the Woody Allen movie that came out of the screen, it is something like that…. One is immersed in a story or a fable* …" the allusion to Allen's film, in which the man of her dreams steps out of the screen and meets the protagonist, indicates that it is a situation where estrangement was present, but in a pleasant unreality.

Something similar when a participant tells how, in the city of Venice, the awareness of living a fantasy is clearer, but this letting go, in a certain way, shows a different level of experience.

We went to a medieval ball in a palace, I walked from morning to night dressed up … *It's like I "got into it" and I was so fascinated. I don't know how to explain it* because when you are in something that you wanted a lot, *it seems like a lie but for me it was natural, I went out in the morning dressed (in the costume) and I stayed like that until the night … I was just one more … I was like a child. … It's the whole environment. I don't know how to explain it. There was no room for anything else … In that sense, I was loose and that's what happened to me, I was loose. … They took you, all of them, by the hand here or there. … I felt like I was in a dream ….*

The possibility of getting lost and being as if in a dream or a story, give the guideline of a form of estrangement in which the notion of reality is not completely lost; however, phrases such as "she was loose", "she was one more", "there was no room for anything else" indicate that it was something more intense, and that she lived a state of estrangement, in an unreality, as a story, theater or dream.

3.2.2.3 Light, illumination, epiphany

In the state of estrangement, in the sensory dimension, the emergence of light takes on particular importance. It emerges in the descriptions: light appears pointing out or configuring aspects of the scene experienced as estrangement. In the aesthetic experience, due to its effects of estrangement, which transforms the lived situation into a stage, light, translucent light, or illumination, acquires a fundamental place, as in the theater. Juan Bautista Ritvo (2010) speaks of the light of *touch: tactile light.* He goes on to say that this light … is "the site par excellence of experience in moments of slumber, of relaxation of bonds, of suffering, of orgasm …" (p. 67). Then, as for illumination, Ritvo relates it to "psychoanalytic light, the light of the unconscious, which returns suddenly on the margins of so-called natural light" (p. 84), and is linked to reflection, rapture and, also, mind fog. We see some of this appearing as, for example, Lacan in Baltimore, in the light of dawn. Gilbert Rose, speaks of the "necessary illusion" that he says covers the experience and is part of this encounter. The aesthetic experience is intimately related to "the apprehension of beauty" which, in the midst of "a certain overwhelming sensation", produces a network of identifications through which one is drawn; according to Meltzer and Harris Williams, as between fluid limits and vanishing edges, like a sort of "enveloping spell", a dream evoked and contained that, in a coming and going, finds its symbolic form. For psychoanalyst and writer Luis Gusmán, light appears as "the instant of lucidity" (p. 41); he affirms that light, linked to lucidity, "appears linked to time in a paradoxical way: as a privileged state, a place to arrive, but at the same time as a threat on the horizon—the ghost of old age—, a good that can be lost" (p. 41), that is, in relation to nostalgia and transience. He relates beauty with splendor, "an aesthetics of splendor, heir to Plotinus' illuminism". And he speaks of "The epiphanization of the object" affirming that in the artist, the privileged, almost evanescent moment when in that "encounter the object is epiphanized, a good encounter, a *coup de dés*" (p. 47). Lucidity is then compared to the pulsating moment, "the privileged moment that Freud gave to the unconscious as the instant in which something of the repressed truth is captured before it closes again; this enables us to think of lucidity … as an epiphanic moment where the subject grazes the sparkle of the truth before the opaque resistance of the discourse hides it again" (p. 51). It is the alteration of perspectival space by that effect of light, the cutout that transforms it into a stage with the irruption of a cutout and a translucence, as in the theater, an appearance in the cutout of background and figure that makes it appear to be something alive, a presence and a sensual materiality. The visual becomes tactile, sensory, and is transferred to a bodily sensation.

As an example, a participant reports about The Taj Mahal, the light through the filigree … the fabulous light, the reflections ….

"Forgive me, he says, the light there is fundamental because the light, at a certain hour, gives you reflections that at other times it doesn't give you …". They recommend you to go at a certain time because that is when the contrasts of the filigree can be seen much more …. The light is defining. The flat surface worked with light reaches a third dimension, it is impressive, it has volume …. It is corporeal. It has a relief … If you put a light in front of it, you don't see the contrast, if you put it to the side, the relief is different. All of that was wonderful for me.

The defining condition of light gives us the guideline of the corporeal and of the pleasure hidden in that estrangement:

> *The reflection in the domes of the mosques* that are farther back and suddenly it is as if they lower the audio and the thing becomes a murmur and it is the light and the colors. It was that instant ... *it was the light, a very particular light*. A certain thing with the aromas too, it was atmospheric ... Something was moving ... to look up, the reflection in a dome, the light ...

The two stories show different aspects of the effect of light, while in the first, it accompanies an atmosphere that creates a scene in which one of the people is immersed and, in the other case, the sudden lighting creates an abrupt cut of the scene and gives the experience something of the ambiguous and disturbing, although both refer to something intensified sensorily, in the order of the marvelous and extraordinary. Something of a tactile and visual order, just as the luminosity predisposes to a state of estrangement, between illusion, reverie, and strangeness. A truth and something linked to the unconscious as apparition.

3.2.3 Entrapment and the "artwork function"

The function of the work of art or, we could say, where art *works* is the dimension of estrangement that manifests itself as being trapped, seduced, or captured by the work. It is an essential part of estrangement, given that this state of being captured, trapped by the work, the situation, the images, is the key to the fact that art is at work. And that we are part of the intensity of that experience. It is expressed as being trapped, entrapped, annihilated, not being able to move, to return, which account for the seductive function of the work and questioning. The work of art as a promoter of an encounter with the real: it is not the subject that contemplates and tries to apprehend the work, but rather the exteriority of the work that grips the subject, as Recalcati et al. (2006) reminds us that Roland Barthes affirms (p. 22). He clarifies that this "being trapped" by the work gives rise, according to Lacan, to a "pleasure of the eye", a pacification of the gaze that has in a sense the effect of the "Apollonian of painting". It has at the same time the picture function in its most radical character, the limit of the possibility of representation of the subject, the subject delivered to the Other's gaze is, "the function in which the subject, has to find himself as such" (p. 24); it summons the *unheimlich*. It is what is insinuated.

Therefore, the "work of art" effect is linked to an entrapment, a form of hypnosis or fascination, something of the suspension of tension that produces relief, overlapping common experience, as happens in experiences in philosophy, religion and art. In the "pacification of the gaze", at the same time, something disturbing is involved. It is what the drive movement between play and repetition accounts for, as well as entrapment in the drive circuit. Fascination and entrapment as part of estrangement imply an active subject who enters some form of interplay with the work, even getting lost and returning to the same place, like the experience referred to by Freud when "lost" in "The Uncanny" (1919). He tells us:

> "Through the empty streets, unknown to me, of a small Italian town, I came to an area whose character I could not doubt for long. I could only see painted women" ... and I hurried to leave the narrow alley turning at the first corner. But ..., suddenly I found myself again in the same street ..., and my hasty departure only resulted in my stopping there for the third time after a new detour. *Then a feeling came over me that I can only describe as ominous,* and I felt joy when, renouncing further voyages of discovery, I found again the Piazza that I had left a short time before.
>
> (Freud, 1919)

As we see, the *unheimlich* is engaged in entrapment, as an aspect of the drive and the ominous, as well as the lived, desired ... the feminine. Thus, the drive and entrapment appear in the description of one of the participants when, in front of Michelangelo's sculptures, she recounts:

> In the case of the stone of these men, the desire to touch, you saw that they tell you "Do not get close to the work ...". It occurred to me to approach, touch and embrace them to get in contact with them. I didn't do it ... You have the impulse. I felt it with the stone men, I would have hugged them or I would have climbed onto them.

The impulse is there, it is of an erotic creative order, to play as a girl too; already in a state of estrangement, she speaks of men, they are not statues.

In the aesthetic experience, estrangement in that form of distancing enables a movement of the drive that accounts for the unconscious desire: not being able to let go, to turn away, to want to touch, to climb. To speak of the tactile dimension in the optical, and the movement of liberation of the drive by "estrangement from reality". It also recovers the space of play, when it is not presented as ominous. It accounts, in the experience of passing from a passive spectator to a participating subject, for the experience that promotes creative acts, in the sense of metaphor, of action even in repetition, and of participation in the configuration of the scene and the work itself, as interpretation. Winnicott argues that the artist's impulse is transferred to the work in creation, that its tension of urgency determines a particular "'discharge" that imposes a certain degree of physical participation (however slight) for the excitement (Winnicott, 1971, p. 119). It is a dynamic tension, which asks not to be resolved—like the paradox—, in order to maintain the eternal contest between the Dionysian and the Apollonian, and a certain relation between thought and non-thought, "of a certain mode of presence of thought in the sensible materiality and of the sense of the insignificant", says Rancière (2009), which constitutes the "aesthetic regime of art" (p. 9).

On the other hand, it is also the condition of the beautiful, in the aesthetic experience, that promotes *metexis*, the participation of the object with the subject. The attraction of the beautiful, Plato's "*metexis*", as part of this experience has the function of a lure, and also has a formative character, as defined by Meltzer in "the apprehension of beauty". However, this "being caught", this "being stung" by the work is not a fall of the subject into the vortex of the Thing, it does not give rise to a Stendhal syndrome. Recalcati et al. (2006) says: "Lacan refers rather to a pleasure of the eye, to being caught by the painting as an aesthetic experience of abandonment, pacification, as a deposition of the gaze".

Nasio (1994) tells us that the work of art hypnotizes the spectator at the same time that it arouses the same creative passion that motivated its creator. The objective—he thinks—is "to numb our conscience to make us permeable to the exterior and interior excitement arising from the contemplated work" (p. 113). This hypnosis in art awakens our creative impulses. And this is what appears in the description of another interviewee, in a drive mode, when he relates having wanted to touch a painting when he was alone in Amsterdam in front of a Vermeer, and he said to himself: "I touch it" [...] "I have it here. This painting I have it here"...

Another example the experience of entrapment is narrated by another person, in which the "alienation" in the midst of a state of estrangement makes him feel directly a character in the story, when he refers to his experience in Rome:

> Il Gesù in Rome ... *I felt like a Jesuit ready to conquer the world for the Holy Catholic Faith and bring the Western world to God the Father*, exaggerating a bit, but that was the feeling. *To enter into that thing so overwhelming and at the same time deeply baroque and at the same time dark* ... and there yes ... in Il Gesù *I remember that a whole world literally grabs you by the eyelashes and starts flipping you over the walls and throws you into the bosom of the kingdom of* ....

We could say that it is almost a state of possession, in which the hypnotic effect alienates him into the situation in a form of non-pathological estrangement, which accounts for the dimension of entrapment and the function of the work of art, in the power of its creative action.

The third moment he remembers with time, almost unwillingly, at the end, since it is the opposite, a situation as he says, ghostly, in which it is the feeling of the unfamiliar that drives him to approach the ominous and almost suffer a fainting spell.

In synthesis, we see in these testimonies how estrangement manifests itself as the core of the aesthetic experience and a condition of possibility. It is a psychic state that refers to a situation between subject and object. The state of estrangement is divided into subcategories that respond to indicators, which are observed in fragments of the story and are related to concepts. There are examples of interviews in which the state of estrangement reveals indicators of several subcategories or dimensions: conditions of unreality, the object's ambiguity, as well as entrapment, which is an effect and condition of estrangement that may be evidenced in various ways. In some accounts, estrangement is evidenced when questions related to the psychic state arise, such as being "dumbfounded", which shows a psychic state that includes something surprising. One testimony speaks of a strangeness that reaches "depersonalization", although it clarifies that it was not pathological; it is the sensation of unreality, or estrangement from the empirical world, which is what defines the sensation of unreality. The scene that is configured ("as if suddenly a kind of scene had been set up") seems more like a scenography, which accounts for the subcategory of the sensation of scenography. It illustrates the condition of the ambiguous object ("a white object floating in the air"), as a dimension that reveals estrangement. It is also the object that traps another interviewee, which expresses the fascination exerted by that object, which becomes ambiguous ("and I don't know what I was looking at because it was extremely simple and flat. I don't know what fascination it held"). The dimension of "entrapment" appears, in "not being able to move the body", or "paralysis", which are two ways of evidencing the entrapment, or capture, by the effect of the work of art, as estrangement. Another manifestation of entrapment is referred to as "not wanting to leave", which also implies a component of desire that begins to come into play. It is a dimension of Eros, which appears in another story when, in the surprise encounter with Santa Maria Novella, he sees her "alone" and recalls the figure of the *fidanzata*. That is, *the bride*.

The temporal dimension, which is part of the manifestation of estrangement and entrapment, and the atmosphere evoked by each subject, varies and is insinuated in this state. Time and concrete reality vanish. The subject of the experience and the Work configure a situation, which is extracted from the daily or the expected future. The expression of **that "thing"** appears a lot in the testimonies, which seems to be directly related to the encounter with the Thing, as Recalcati says, in the line of the category of the ambiguous object, as defined by Oliveras quoting Valéry. A finding emerges from the interviews, which is the dimension of light. The weighting and highlighting of the effect of light contributes to the observation of the ambiguous object, which appears either as illuminated by a "divine ray", "something bright" or "something white". It also emerges as that which floods a scene, creating an atmosphere, like a faint light that colors the dusk of a scene, described by another interviewee, in which domes and cats' glow at dusk. One is reminded of the scene described by Lacan, when he states that the unconscious "is Baltimore at dawn", with its complexity of light effects. This is highlighted by another testimony, when the interviewee recounts feeling taken by her account of the Taj Majal, in which "the light is defining". In my fieldwork, a luminous dimension emerges, related to the effects of estrangement, both pleasant, as a relaxation of the ties with the conscious, and also as illuminating a scene, or as a clarification, in the emergence of an unconscious truth that can be thought on the basis of the continuity of the story, the associations and metaphors used to describe what was experienced. The light approaches the effect of estrangement, as Ritvo says, states of sleepiness in the description of sensations, where the light is defining, transporting people to another dimension, which seems to be a sensual component. We see how estrangement opens to the dimension of the possibility of illusion, not only as fantasy, but as the condition of possibility of another scene linked to something of reality, which is the object of art and the construction of an experience in which one is participating. The screen of representation, in these conditions of estrangement, becomes permeable and what seemed fantastic becomes real; it appears as if the screen were opened, in an unimaginable dimension. These situations can become marvelous or ominous, as Freud says. In a less blunt way, like having entered a dream or a fairy tale, refers an interviewee when she "enters" and "lets herself go". The screen is torn, but not broken, it is opened or permeabilized, we could say, so that in the estrangement something of the alien or strange can appear and be appropriated, and something of the alien of the world can be metabolized; it is the possibility of playing, in a certain way in the zone of illusion, being an adult, in an experience with art, and "losing oneself" in the estrangement as an aesthetic experience. The state of reverie, between dream and fantasy, is enabled in the estrangement in the aesthetic experience, and appears as in a trance. At another extreme, another participant says that he cannot believe what he sees, as happens to Freud on the Acropolis. He too cannot believe what he sees. "This is not real." Entrapment, or what we call artwork function, is something that is the essence of estrangement, hypnosis, or dream states, seduction; getting caught up, being caught or lost, not wanting to move, define the way of living the edges of experience. It is something rather disturbing or something in the order of pleasure that one does not want to leave. In all cases, it is about the drive enclave where this dimension of estrangement happens: the impulse to touch, the paralysis, and the not moving referred to in several testimonies, or an indefinable state as reported by another, that alludes to something of love and nostalgia. Between the physical and the drive, passion circulates in different ways, between disavowal and playing, the drive emerges, generally sublimated, but also, in the encounter, the evocative and complex power of the lost object is found again as the lost or as a surprising finding, which coincides with pleasure, and something of repetition, which in a beyond, pulsates something elaborative. The dark object at its extreme point is the hole, which as emptiness left by the thing, generates anguish but also demands a new alternative to find again in non-pathological estrangement the coordinates of pleasure where something of its own is built, expropriated from the strangeness of the world.

3.3 Modes of pleasure

3.3.1 Paradoxical pleasure

Strangeness as the nerve center of the aesthetic experience triggers complex modes of pleasure. The state of estrangement, by its very ambiguous nature of blurred edges, accounts for sensations that move the body and produce modes of feeling—modes of pleasure—which, as a correlate of estrangement, is a paradoxical pleasure. Paradoxical pleasure configures this category that, in the interweave of the interviews with the theoretical framework, reveals gradations and modes that approach a positive pleasure, as something mystical, or an "epiphany" and a "negative" pleasure, a pleasure with pain, such as nostalgia (*Nostos*, "return", and *algia*, "pain"), or ominous feelings, some disturbing form of extreme feeling of living estrangement in the aesthetic experience. Paradoxical pleasure, therefore, is a mode of pleasure, a correlate and formalization of estrangement, which accounts for this combinatory that entails modes that appear to be in opposition. However, if it is assumed that in the aesthetic experience (as estrangement), the experience of the beautiful and also of the sinister, the Apollonian and the Dionysian is involved, it can be understood why the pleasure that arises is a paradoxical pleasure.

The strong idea of this category determines that pleasure in estrangement as an aesthetic experience, is a "paradoxical pleasure" that promotes a sensation of varied qualities and intensities, modes of pleasure *and beyond*, whose condition is to move the subject in such a way that it touches the unconscious, constituting that paradox in the effective condition of the aesthetic experience. The point at which sensation transfigures the original, which gives way to a drive movement in the sense of Eros, as a ligature or articulation. This form of pleasure manifests itself in a psyche-soma movement that *touches* the unconscious, and results in an experience in the order of the event. It is proposed that an aesthetic experience takes on its full potency as a creative effect. The aesthetic experience, in the *estrangement*, produces modes of pleasure specific to the experience with art. This is what we understand as a modern aesthetic experience, insofar as the beautiful does not acquire its full potency without that which subverts it or contains the *pathos* of the Dionysian in the middle and, at the same time, the veil of the Apollonian. Trías says that "nevertheless the beautiful, in order to preserve its aesthetic force, must be in relation to the real; beauty is an Apollonian veil that must make us sense the Dionysian chaos that pulsates in it"; for this author, "there can be no aesthetic effect without the sinister being, in some way, present in the artistic work" (quoted by Recalcati et al. 2006), however, it must be present in the form of absence, it must be veiled, which gives the work "its magic, mystery and fascination". In this line, Freud says, in "The Ominous" quoting Schelling: "Veil the divine and surround it with a certain *Unheimlichkeit*, mystery". This paradox constitutes the "aesthetic regime of art" that Rancière defines, in which there is dynamic tension that demands not to be resolved in order to maintain the eternal competition between the Dionysian and the Apollonian and the presence of a certain mode of "thought in sensible materiality". This dynamic tension that demands not to be resolved is, in psychoanalysis, Winnicott's plea in relation to paradox as a possibility of construction of creative subjectivity, in "paradoxical thinking between "rationality and primary creativity", as Raquel Zak de Goldstein (2012) calls it.

The mode of pleasure that makes art possible, according to Jauss, must be investigated since the attitude of enjoyment, which triggers and makes art possible, is the "primordial aesthetic experience"; it cannot be excluded, but must become again the object of theoretical reflection, as stated by (Jauss, 2002, p. 31) He said that primordial aesthetic experience, implies a pleasure different from the pleasure of the senses and that "...Only Freud,...recovered, integrating it into his theory" states Carballal (2014, p. 69). What kind of pleasure are we talking about, beyond the aesthetic, promoted by art? What is the deep dimension that unfolds in art? And what is its relation with the sexual? In this regard, Freud wonders how is it that "...many things which, if they were real, would not give pleasure... can become sources of pleasure for the poet's audience and spectators" (Freud, 1908). What is this plus that is added, and only by which the work of art becomes what it is? (Gadamer, 1998, p. 20).

This enigmatic question involving something that promotes pleasure and something that implies a plus, is what questions Freud before the Acropolis when he is astonished to disprove what he sees and says, "Such disbelief is evidently an attempt to disavow a fragment of objective reality, but in it there is something strange," and continues, why such disbelief regarding something that, on the contrary, *promises high pleasure?* Truly paradoxical behavior!" Art's promise of pleasure, as well as its roots in the sexual repressed, are the Freudian foundations of pleasure and its complex relation with infantile desire. Promise as a mode of "forepleasure," which is, paradoxically, an "overpowering" shock, disorienting to the point of disbelief. How do we account for this complex, combined mode of pleasure?

[...] the initial metaphorization is taking steps around pleasure and reality... which always seems to oscillate between more than two logics ... an oscillation stabilized in the intimacy of the "tertiary processes", which give us a surprising power: "paradoxical thinking" (Zak de Goldstein, 2012).

We call paradoxical or ambiguous this mode of pleasure that runs through a range of expressions, from the marvelous to the ominous in different forms of presentation that produce a sensory shock, a "thinking sensoriality" that involves the *real*, the body and the emergence of the unconscious. The pleasure of art, says Freud in "The Discomfort of Culture", provides a "weak narcosis" and although "the enjoyment of beauty is accompanied by a particular sensation with a soft intoxicating effect", "it does not move our corporeality".

At the same time, Freud affirms that the pleasure intimately related to beauty derives from the sexual, as a mode of pleasure called ultimate pleasure, which comes from sexual love. Freud says, "one of the forms of manifestation of love, sexual love, (which) has procured for us the most intense experience of overwhelming pleasurable sensation, thus giving us the archetype for our aspiration to bliss". Meanwhile, Nasio (2015) refers the effect of art to beauty, but recognizes that "beauty is not an idea but a feeling and even a physical sensation, something we feel with our whole body" (p. 113) and that it promotes, in that effect that touches and surprises the subject, the manifestation of a positive poetics of the unconscious.

It is proposed to think pleasure in the aesthetic experience as a pleasure that sets the psyche in motion, insofar as it touches the originary. Its origin, in the experience of satisfaction, refers to traces of pleasure that touch the body (real, original). This characteristic of pleasure in estrangement is referred to as "sensation", for which words are not enough. If the aesthetic experience "touches" the subject, it is because something in his unconscious is being moved. This would be the allegory. The Freudian unconscious, Rancière (2009) proposes, is constituted in the "aesthetic unconscious", a sphere of privileged effectiveness of art where *pathos*, as an encounter with the sensitive matter of the body itself and of the work, is what accounts for the disturbing and at the same time for a tension that promotes other forms of creativity. Jauss understands *Poiesis* as "poetic capacity"; it is the experience in which "man *manages to meet the world*" (Jauss, 2002).

Double and paradoxical, the aesthetic experience in its metaphorizing potential in a dynamic reading accounts for processes called "tertiary", which circulate in a "between" reality and pleasure that involves creative processes, as Fiorini (2006) explains.

3.3.2 Genuss, pleasure, and symbolic phenomena

In modern aesthetics, it is Jauss who recovers the question of the term enjoyment in aesthetic experience by saying that the old-fashioned usage *geniessen*, "enjoy", produces a prejudice and states that "if we consider aesthetic experience more closely, aesthetic enjoyment is distinguished from simple sensory pleasure, as almost unanimously confirmed by all aesthetic theories since the Kantian doctrine of disinterested satisfaction..." (Jauss, 2002, p. 40). Now, we know that the term "pleasure" alludes to "sensation" in several variants. To a sensory experience. In aesthetics, the sensation of pleasure is linked to the etymology of the discipline, "*Aisthesis*", "sensation" or the "sensitive" from its very core of existence when it emerges as a universe with autonomy in the philosophy of the 18th century. Thus, it establishes relations with the beautiful, the good, the desirable or the "good form", which produces the sensation of pleasure, as an experience with art or the beautiful. Kant determines this difference, this pleasure linked to the beautiful; what is linked to what is beyond the beautiful, he calls "the sublime": the forces that overflow the form are in relation to a feeling that is of awe or respect rather than pleasure. From the theorization of Kant and the post-Kantians, and the citizenship card of aesthetics with Baumgarten, conceptualizations that underpin sensation with reason, or some form of knowledge, are included. Rancière says that "aesthetics is the name of the category that, for two centuries, has designated in the West the sensitive fabric and the form of intelligibility of what we call 'art', as a specific form of experience since the eighteenth century in the West" (2013, p. 9).

In psychoanalysis, pleasure implies a concept that refers to the pleasure principle: that which sets the psychic apparatus in motion; it is one of the two principles of mental functioning, which in the first place aims at avoiding displeasure. It appears at the beginning of psychic life, starting from what Freud called the "experience of satisfaction", which later gives rise to the forms of desire and pleasure, setting in motion the psyche and the thread of thinking and desiring. This inaugural situation highlights the place of pleasure, which underpins the construction of the psyche, between a primitive real Ego, a pure pleasure Ego and a definitive reality Ego. The principle of pleasure is opposed to the principle of reality, which in psychoanalytic theory makes psychic dynamics work, in the sense of desire and culture. But in relation to art, these principles, rather than opposing each other, seem to establish a particular exchange in which reality is placed in suspense, outside of pathology. This suspension of the tensions of reality, as Winnicott affirms, produces relief and, it is proposed, pleasure. In relation to art, Freud pronounces himself on the basis of a type of pleasure that he calls previous pleasure. Although he recognizes a deeper pleasure, in the manner of catharsis, which will be genuine pleasure, how does Freud understand this economy of pleasure, and what are the characteristics of art as a mode of pleasure? How does art make us feel "a high pleasure, which probably has tributaries from various sources", as Freud asks himself in 1907? The model of the poet points the way by which such pleasure takes place, for through the "authentic *ars poetica*," which "tempers the character of daydreaming ... and bribes us by means of a purely formal, i.e., aesthetic, gain of pleasure ...," we "feel a high pleasure" by lifting the barriers of repression and producing pleasure instead of scandal, Freud states in "The Creative Writer and the Day-dreaming." Then he determines that: "We call this gain of pleasure that is offered to us in order to make possible with it the detachment of a greater pleasure, coming from psychic sources situated at a greater depth, the incentive premium or previous pleasure".[1]

Freud then defines that all aesthetic pleasure has the character of that previous pleasure, and that "genuine jouissance" arises from the "liberation of tensions in the interior of our soul", as the model of aesthetic pleasure, and understands that "here we would be at the doors of new, interesting and complex inquiries ...". Freud is outlining an investigation in which pleasure or aesthetic enjoyment is pleasure that through the pleasure premium, previous pleasure, muffled, generates expectation and seduces to achieve the loosening of repression and inhibitions, to achieve a final pleasure that would account for discharges in the manner of Aristotelian catharsis, where sexual pleasure is involved as a discharge of excitations, relief of tensions in relation to forbidden or repressed fantasies that access a form of "consciousness with pleasure".

Play is an essential aspect of aesthetic enjoyment. On the other hand, Gadamer clarifies that play "means, at the same time, that playing always demands a 'playing-with" (1993, p. 69). "There is nothing other than *participatio*, the inner participation in that movement that repeats itself" (p. 73). He explains that every work leaves to the one who receives it a space of play that he has to fill. It is an active movement that involves the subject of the experience in a continuous "being-active-with". It is this participation, being active *with* in this "play" that relieves and summons tensions, repeats and works through, that characterizes the aesthetic experience, as proposed, and engages something of participation in the phenomenon of estrangement. It is proposed, under these conditions, that paradoxical pleasure happens at the same time and is superimposed in different modes, giving rise to something like previous pleasure and a mode of final pleasure, which includes a shock effect that is what accounts for the emergence of the unconscious.

In this sense, we understand the point in which Freudian research shows that pleasure as a psychic engine does not seem to be the only mode of psychic economy: there is a beyond pleasure, which Freud relates to concepts that provide a conceptual twist in which the pair of pleasure-unpleasure becomes other terms that are Eros and Thanatos. It will be the repetition and the link or not of the drive that insists, something also summoned in the encounter with art, in estrangement as an aesthetic experience where the pain of tragedy, feared phantasms and forbidden desires have a privileged field of experience. There, a beyond pleasure emerges that is part of paradoxical pleasure as an experience that happens, occurs and somehow promotes the repetition or actualization of something lost, which is the mark of a trace but with a predominance of Eros as coordinates of pleasure, which leaves the lost object, and summons the encounter with the object of art, in the midst of a strange feeling of being "lost" in the aesthetic experience.

Following Freud, it is understood that art in its relation to the beautiful has its roots in sexual arousal, beyond the beauty or not of the genitals, in a promise of pleasure from something that is seen. It is felt in the whole body, as psyche-soma and subject. In the extension of Freud's work in questioning in relation to aesthetics, clues appear to know that pleasure is not only linked to something beautiful, as Freud enunciates and interrogates it in his liminal article, "The Uncanny". In "disturbing strangeness", something that transcends the beautiful also moves in relation to art and aesthetics: the strange, the hidden, that which returns from time immemorial, the forbidden, the ominous. Modes of aesthetic enjoyment interrogate the subject in estrangement. Although Freud postulates that it is very rare for the psychoanalyst to dedicate himself to aesthetic inquiries, it may happen that in some situations he becomes interested in "some of these strange qualities, such as the 'ominous'", says Freud in "the uncanny". In that same text, Freud inaugurates a modern way of thinking about aesthetics and gives an account of that which, beyond the beautiful, shakes aesthetics and its experience, exposing the complex relationship between the strange and the familiar, the beautiful and the sinister, producing in psychoanalytic research what Trias emphasizes as the consequences of the reflection of Kantian aesthetics, from which "the beautiful and the sublime are synthesized in a single category, in which the sensible datum (and its limitation) and the infinite spirit enter into connection" (Trias, 2001). What is the psychoanalytic correlate of this conceptualization?

3.3.3 *The ominous, the mystical and a "Sensible Epiphany"*

One of the modes of pleasure appears in reaction to an object that promotes an auratic dimension, which is the encounter with the lost object, with what appears as presence-absence of the lost object, which is underpinned in the Freudian ominous and accounts for a complex and profound relation between the sublime and the ominous, and the relation between forms of sublimated, "muffled" spiritual pleasure and the repressed or split component in the ominous, as the forbidden or the divine that must remain hidden or secret. The Freudian ominous thus constitutes the cornerstone of contemporary aesthetics, insofar as it relates the notion of "sensation" to something beyond the senses, which Aesthetics as the "science of the beautiful" is unable to explain. He refers that he uses the linguistic term "sensation" laxly to allude to sensations of mental mirages, such as estrangement. Freud says:

> We must also include1 in the category of the miraculous and the 'uncanny' the peculiar feeling we have, in certain moments and situations, of having had exactly the same experience once before or of having once before been in the same place, though our efforts never succeed in clearly remembering the previous occasion that announces itself in this way"… I am aware that I am merely following loose linguistic usage when I call what arises in a person at such moments a 'feeling'. What is no doubt in question is a judgement, and, more precisely, a perceptual judgement; but these cases have nevertheless a character quite of their own, and we must not leave out of account the fact that what is looked for is never remembered.
>
> (Freud, 1901, p. 265)

The encounter with the lost or forgotten appears as something marvelous and sublime in its relation with the Freudian uncanny, as developed by Trías (2001), who affirms that the beautiful and the sublime are synthesized in a dimension together with the sinister, which is what gives vitality to the work; the sensitive and "the infinite spirit enter into connection. Beauty will be divine presence, incarnation, revelation of the infinite in the finite" (Trias quote by Recalcati et al., 2006). This way of defining the experience and the relation with pleasure is what one of the interviewees relates, when she was in the Sistine Chapel in front of Michelangelo's paintings, and refers:

> ... I am close to something that is immeasurable, that's why I use the word "astounding". I felt in front of something majestic and masterful, very big, and it gave me pleasure to be close to that painting or those extraordinary sculptures. There is something "extraordinary" and masterful about it.
>
> When they talk about mystics, they say they have this feeling of "elevation" or "contact with everything". I don't want to use the word God because it seems a little strong to me ... Something mystical. In the Sistine Chapel it was something mystical, I reached mystical pleasure.

Another participant also describes his experience at the Mayan ruins, saying:

> It seemed to me that it connected me with something that exceeded geography and connected me with history. Time and space came together and that moved me, it was stronger than me, tears were falling at that moment ... It is those moments when something bursts in and makes you cry, in this case it was not of sadness but of emotion before such a wonderful thing. ...Magnanimous.

Terms with which one seeks to describe something of the lived experience, something that surpasses it, something "grandiose" and makes him live an "infinite" or extraordinary situation, or the marvelous, which is what defines the Kantian sublime, following Trías. It is what Alberto goes on to describe as "a marvelous situation": "The sensation was something rare. Rare and marvelous ...", which accounts for what Trías describes as "initiation, the starting point of a journey and voyage towards the very heart of the divine ..." and towards the mysteriousness of the origins, which produces upon its revelation, at the same time as the marvelous, "the *feeling* of the ominous". This accounts for the variants of the ominous in Freud's *das Unheimlich,* whose very definition points to a paradoxical significance that will force us to understand, in this sense, that "*Unheimlich* and *Heimlich* come to mean the same thing: the mysterious, hidden and secret", as Trías (2001) affirms. This is what the participant himself describes as his first aesthetic experience:

> My first experience with the images of art or painting allude to something solitary, mysterious, concentrated, a little secret too, right? There was something secret … It was a mysterious painting, everything was mysterious. It contained all that mysterious atmosphere.

Now, if we follow the Freudian reasoning, to which Trías' conjecture is added, we find definitions that swing between the marvelous, the sublime, the mystical and… the ominous, given that the mode of pleasure is described, in that something of the sexual origin of pleasure, forbidden, is related to a pleasure, in the order of the marvelous and the strange, which he proposes to call "sensitive epiphany".

He refers to an account of Michelangelo's Pietà: "I was left with a very strange sensation; it was a wonderful situation as if the gates of heaven had suddenly opened".

In another way, another interviewee refers: "In [the church] Il Gesù I remember that a whole world literally grabs you by the eyelashes and starts flipping you over the walls and throws you into the bosom of the kingdom of heaven".

It is understood that the terms used point to the alienating threshold between the bodily and the rational, that "the gates of heaven" and its correlate with "the gateway" to the place where we all have dwelt at the beginning of life, account for an experience, as Freud says, which refers to something of the ominous, as well as longing for something of the lost, the maternal womb, female genitalia, the lost part of oneself, for which he defines "the ominous is the door of access to the ancient site of the infant, to the place in which each one of us has dwelt at the beginning". Therefore, the ominous is "the once domestic, the familiar of old… reanimated by an impression". As happens in the aesthetic experience, it engages nostalgia for something lost and says "Love is nostalgia", longing that activates the encounter with art in the aesthetic experience. This is what defines the auratic dimension of the object and describes that experience.

3.3.3.1 Aura and nostalgia

It is proposed that this auratic dimension is described as either nostalgic or mystical, given that, as defined by Walter Benjamin, the *aura* (and its loss) in the work of art is "the unrepeatable manifestation of a remoteness". This remoteness is nostalgic, and accounts for the loss of the cultural value that the work of art had in its origin, that is to say, of religious worship, a place lost in the modern aesthetic experience. However, I propose that the aesthetic experience, in some way, reintroduces something of the aura as a dimension that promotes the aesthetic experience in "The instant of lucidity", according to Gusmán (2010), for whom, as we mentioned above, "lucidity appears paradoxically linked to time:

as a privileged state, a place to arrive, but at the same time as a threat on the horizon -the ghost of old age-, a good that can be lost". Cultural value emerges as what this author calls "the epiphanization of the object" (Gusmán, 2010, p. 128). As we have said, for Gusmán, this instant of lucidity is compared to the pulsating moment, "the privileged moment that Freud granted to the unconscious as the instant in which something of the repressed truth is captured before it closes again, whichenables us to think of lucidity as an epiphanic moment when the subject brushes against the sparkle of truth before the opaque resistance of discourse hides it again" (p. 51). In this line, I affirm that there were times when the self is not self, ancient present times when an unconscious reality is touched and, as an instantaneous vision, a truth is discovered in consciousness, something of primordial times. Therefore, both aesthetic experience and psychoanalytic experience involve the possibility of experiencing a truth.

From another point of reflection, the sensory and bodily dimension that promotes the aesthetic experience shows its most original nature, which derives from the *substance* of "primary creativity", "which is supposed to be more fundamental than the sublimation of drives", and is, says Winnicott in *Reality and Play* (1971), "the nostalgia for an immediacy that cancels the distancing necessarily introduced by representation".

The nostalgia that accompanies the dimension of the lost object, or experiences approaching the mystical, account for the auratic dimension. They produce the same feeling of helplessness and ominousness. Something of the *spectral,* which emerges in contemporary aesthetic experience, for Hal Foster (2001), would be an *elaborate* way of seeking to "connect the lost spaces of childhood". This nostalgia, pain with pleasure, *nostalgia,* is what one of the participants of the study describes when, in the experience with Muek's sculptures, he relates this sensation in the order of pleasure:

> ... but an immersion in an original situation. In a very large space in Proa, I had a couple of old men on the beach, huge figures with huge umbrellas and with a kind of relationship of contact between them, a very complex mixture of feelings that communicated it. That is a work in which I immersed myself, isn't it? You could see the kind of contact of the masterfully made bodies, and it conveyed an impressive complexity of feelings in that room. Everything has a point of helplessness ... It is something that awakens nostalgia ..., let's say a softly painful memory. *Nostos,* where nostalgia comes from, means pain for the lost place ... Something like an unspeakable remoteness ... Yes, I mean it was a very indescribable mixture; there was warmth, there was tenderness, there was boredom, there was abandonment, the extraordinary thing about it was the complexity of the feelings that it communicated.

The atmosphere of longing also appears, as Foster says, in seeking to "connect the lost spaces of childhood" in what another interviewee describes as his first aesthetic experience, with a picture painted by his grandfather, which was a sailboat at sea:

> My first experience with the images of art or painting allude to something solitary, mysterious, concentrated, a little secret too, right? There was something secret?

It was a mysterious painting, everything was mysterious. It contained all that mysterious atmosphere… it was something that didn't come from that side, it was something that belonged to my grandfather and it was that: mystery, solitude, remoteness. That's my first aesthetic experience. Rarity. I always thought that images with a strong melancholic meaning are the most attractive, maybe because melancholic images are the most lasting, I think there is something about that, isn't there, the temporality of melancholy in the image is greater.

Benjamin (1973) speaks of the aura, stating: "What is the aura properly speaking? A particular weft of space and time: the unrepeatable appearance of a remoteness, however close it may be found". The work of art reproduces a link with the distant that has been secularized and, at the same time, emptied of its original meaning. The work of art becomes so in a museum to the extent that it is stripped of its here and now: the site of an ancient statue of the goddess Venus, Benjamin says, placed among the Greeks who made her an object of worship, is the temple. Another is the location of the same statue given by medieval clerics, "but both were confronted in the same way with its unrepeatability, in other words, with its aura". The original way of integrating the work of art in the context of tradition undoubtedly found its expression within the cult. Thus, the most ancient works of art were born, as we know, in the service of a ritual that was first magical and, in a second time, religious. But it is of decisive importance that this auratic mode of existence of the work of art is never entirely detached from its ritual function. In other words: the unique value of the "authentic" work of art is always, in any case, theologically founded. This foundation can be mediated as much as you like, but it is still recognizable to us as secularized ritual, even in the most profane forms of the cult of beauty …", explains Benjamin (p. 36). In this seeing and being seen from the auratic dimension, it is necessary to recover the potential of erotic evocation of pleasure at stake.

The complexity of this mode of pleasure emerges in relation to play and to a primary "sensation" of pleasure related to the lifting of repression by the work of art in the state of estrangement and reverie. In this place, tensions are relieved and the suppression inherent to the reality principle is suspended in favor of an experience of pleasure, which we must not disregard, however slight it may be.

Note

1 N.A: This theory of the "incentive premium" and of "prior pleasure" was applied by Freud to the joke in the book he devoted to it (1905). The nature of "prior pleasure" was also examined in *Three Essays on Sexual Theory*.

References

Adorno, Th. W. (1970/2004) Teoría estética, Madrid, Ediciones Akal, p. 113

Aulagnier, P. (1997/1977) La violencia de la interpretación; del pictograma al Enunciado, Amorrortu, Buenos Aires, 1997

Badiou, A. (2000a) El ser y el acontecimiento, Buenos Aires, Manantial, p. 6.

Badiou, A. (2000b) Presentación de la edición en castellano de El ser y el acontecimiento. Acontecimiento, 10(19–20), 11–25.

Benjamin, W. (1973) "La obra del arte en la época de la reproductibilidad técnica" en Discursos interrumpidos I, técnica, Madrid, Taurus, pp. 17–33

Benyakar, M. (2000) "Lo traumático y lo ominoso". Cuestionamientos Teórico-Clínicos acerca del procesamiento de las amenazas. Simposio Preparatorio de las Jornadas Trauma – Duelo – Cuerpo. Dpto. de Niños y Psicosomática. Asociación Psicoanalítica Argentina (A.P.A.) 23 de Mayo del.

Carballal, R. (2014) No-organicidad en la obra de arte moderna: collage, montaje y alegoría. Tesis Doctoral (UDELAR).

Deleuze, G. (1991) Una ontología de lo posible. In Conferencia leída en el Museo Sofía Imber, Caracas, el (Vol. 24).

Fiorini, H. (2006) "El psiquismo creador", en Teoría y clínica de los procesos terciario, Buenos Aires, Nueva Visión.

Foster, H. (2001) "El retorno de lo real", en La vanguardia a finales del siglo, Akal, Madrid.

Freud, S. (1901) "The Psychopathology of Everyday Life: Forgetting, Slips of the Tongue, Bungled Actions, Superstitions and Errors", in The Standard Edition of the Complete Psychological Works of Sigmund Freud, London, Hogarth Press and the Institute of Psycho-analysis.

Freud, S. (1908) "Creative Writers and Day-Dreaming", in The Standard Edition of the Complete Psychological Works of Sigmund Freud, London, Hogarth Press and the Institute of Psycho-analysis, pp. 141–154.

Freud, S. (1919) "The 'Uncanny'", in The Standard Edition of the Complete Psychological Works of Sigmund Freud, London, Hogarth Press and the Institute of Psycho-analysis, pp. 217–256.

Freud, S. (1936) "A Disturbance of Memory on the Acropolis", in The Standard Edition of the Complete Psychological Works of Sigmund Freud, London, Hogarth Press and the Institute of Psycho-analysis, pp. 237–248.

Freud, S. (1899) "Sobre los recuerdos encubridores", in Obras completas, Vol. III, Buenos Aires, Amorrortu, p. 310.

Gadamer, H. G. (1993) Verdad y método. Fundamentos de una hermenéutica filosófica, HERMENEIA 7, Quinta Edición. Ediciones Sígueme – Salamanca.

Gadamer, H. G. (1998) La Actualidad De Lo Bello, Argentina, Paidós ibérica.

Goldstein, G. (2005) La experiencia estética, Buenos Aires, del estante editorial.

Green, A. (1995) La metapsicologia revisitada, Buenos Aires, Editorial Eudeba.

Gusmán, L. (2010) "El instante de lucidez", in Conjetural N° 53, Buenos Aires, Ediciones Sitio, p. 51.

Huxley, A. (1956/2009) Las puertas de la percepción. Cielo e infierno, Traducción de Miguel de Hernani, Barcelona, Editorial Edhasa. ISBN 978-84-350-1860-9.

Jauss, H. R. (2002) Pequeña apología de la experiencia estética, Buenos Aires/Barcelona, Paidós, p. 35.

Lacan, J. (2006) "El sujeto y el otro: la alienación", en El seminario de Jacques Lacan. Libro 11, Los cuatro conceptos fundamentales del psicoanálisis, cap. XVI, Buenos Aires, Paidós.

Laurent, E. (2003) "Ciudades psicoanalíticas", Virtualia No 8, June-July.

Mannoni, O. (1973) La otra escena. Claves de lo imaginario, Buenos Aires, Amorrortu, p. 8.

Nasio, J. D. (1994) "El magnífico niño del Psicoanálisis", en El concepto de sujeto y objeto en la teoría de Jacques Lacan. Barcelona, Gedisa.

Nasio, J. D. (2015) Arte y psicoanálisis, Buenos Aires, Paidós, p. 135.

Oliveras, E. (2005) Theory of the ambiguous object in contemporary art. Revista Espacios, pp. 92–97. http://documents.tips/documents/teoria-del-objeto-ambiguo.html

Perniola, M. (2001) "Le ultime correnti dell'estetica in Italia", en Nino Borsellino y Lucio Felici: Storia della letteratura italiana. Il Novecento. Scenari di fine secolo, Milán, Garzanti.

Ranciere, J. (2009) The Aesthetic Unconscious, Translated by Debra Keates and James Swenson, Cambridge, Polity.

Recalcati, M., Brousse, M.-H., Wajcman, G., Coccoz, V., Giner Ponce, X, Vinciperra, R-P. (2006) Las tres estéticas de Lacan, Buenos Aires, Ediciones El Cifrado.

Rella, F. (1981) "El silencio y las palabras", en El pensamiento en tiempos de crisis, Barcelona, Paidós.

Ritvo, J. B. (2010) "Erotica de la luz: astillas de luz, fragmentos de goce", in Revista Conjetural, N° 53, September, p. 67.

Rose, G. J. (1992/1980) The Power of Form, Nueva York, International Universities Press.

Rosolato, G. (1978) La relación de desconocido, Madrid, Ediciones Petrel.

Trías, E. (2001) Lo bello y lo siniestro, Barcelona, Ariel.

Winnicott, D. (1971/1998) Realidad y juego, Barcelona, Gedisa.

Zak de Goldstein, R. (2012) Personal communication and unpublished writing.

Zukerfeld, R. (2002) "Psicoanálisis, vulnerabilidad somática y resiliencia." IV Congreso Argentino de Psicoanálisis, Rosario, mayo de 2002.

4 Destinies and Estrangements

Hysteria, Narcissism, and Melancholia

4.1 The "Stendhal syndrome", disturbed estrangement

In the field of psychiatry, Graziella Magherini is a relevant author for her research on the aesthetic experience. Investigating the subjective impact of aesthetic experience, some authors have focused on the disturbing and disorganizing potential of aesthetic experience. Magherini in 1990 coined the term *Stendhal syndrome* for a series of sudden attacks of acute psychic suffering lasting from a few hours to a few days, observed and studied in the 1980s in tourists and visitors to Florence who were interested in art. These subjects, who later became patients, had been in good physical and psychic condition when they left their home to undertake the trip. The symptoms or phenomena could be awakened for the first time in a hotel room, in a museum or church, or simply in the street, where so many ancient monumental palaces overshadow the visitor in Florence.

The crises ranged from panic attacks with strong physical discomfort and therefore with fear of fainting, suffocation, of dying or going mad, vertigo, tachycardia, as well as a need to be with a loved one or relative; or else, episodes of depression with a sudden compulsion to return home; in some cases, even an intense sense of alienation, with the extreme and unpleasant feeling that the surrounding world had become hostile or a threat. In other words, the author encountered a set of factors whose interaction led to a real crisis and, in many cases, hospitalization.

These situations are considered an interplay between factors intrinsic and extrinsic to the subject, where the psychopathological production was the product of the confluence of several factors, none of which alone would be capable of precipitating it; these are considered as risk factors.

In psychiatric terms, these are often acute psychotic reactions, generally experienced by foreigners visiting Florence, and can be classified as brief atypical forms. But one constant emerges: an identity crisis and, therefore, of the cohesion of the *Self*, derived from the concatenation of personal history, travel, and the impact of art; it may develop at various levels, from the paraconfusional oneiroid to the more strictly psychotic, or the depersonalization associated with panic attacks. When more detailed observation

DOI: 10.4324/9781003591559-5

was possible, the author was able to detect the rupture of an equilibrium in which the *splitting* mechanism was the most dominant. The onset of the crisis seemed to form a process of change in the personality in which a heightened awareness of the self and of reality is foreshadowed.

From a psychopathological point of view, the developments of Magherini on the "Stendhal syndrome" (Magherini) and the "Jerusalem syndrome" (Bar-El) point to the description of cases where the phenomenon that gathers some of these characteristics and others, such as experiences of epiphanies, or loss of the spatial-temporal notion, loss of the notion of self, up to the extreme of passionate infatuation with the victim's kidnapper ("Stockholm syndrome"), or a sudden and radical spiritual transformation, but they become pathological (Magherini, 1990). Up to this point, these experiences with art or aesthetic and spiritual experiences have been studied.

The author believes that this observed phenomenon has been most evident in Florence because it is a city with a high concentration of works of art; it is "a great showcase of the past, presenting an exceptionally long and intense history, a place frequented by historical presences and memories" (p. 171).

Being a devoted reader of Stendhal, the author observed that the cases presented to her in Florence reminded her of those adolescent readings of Stendhal, who renewed in his time the fashion of traveling and recounting his journeys. She recalled a passage of this writer's where he recounted a journey of 1817 that included Rome, Naples, and Florence. In it, Stendhal writes that when *descending from the Apennines towards Florence* his heart begun to pound*: there lived Dante, Michelangelo, Leonardo Da Vinci.* Stendhal continues, "I had so often seen many scenes of Florence that I knew it beforehand; I was able to move about without a guide" (Magherini, 1990, p. 176).

When visiting Santa Croce in Florence, Stendhal (2017) tells us that there, inside the church, where he was left alone, kneeling before the pulpit, he feels "... enraptured by the beauty of the Sibyl of Volterrano" (p. 17).

> I was already in a sort of ecstasy at the thought of being in Florence and at the nearness of the great men whose tombs I had just seen. Absorbed in the contemplation of sublime beauty, I saw it up close, I touched it, so to speak. I had reached that point of emotion where celestial sensations inspired by the fine arts and passionate feelings meet. Leaving the Santa Croce my heart was pounding; I felt what in Berlin they call nerves; life was draining out of me and I walked fearful of falling.
>
> (p. 21)

Magherini explains that the choice of the name "Stendhal syndrome" was not only due to the disturbance that the author relates in his visit to

Santa Croce, but also to the life and personality of this man, who was open to emotional experiences to the point of becoming a paradigm of this predisposition. Stendhal writes his diaries conveying the psychological tension resulting from the impressions gathered during his travels. What Stendhal seeks in an art object is more its vitality than its history or its erudite mystique.

Stendhal's experience in Santa Croce reminded the author of what happened to Freud at the Acropolis, one of the most transcendent emotional experiences he had—as described in the open letter to Romain Rolland—which touched oedipal founts.

This phenomenon described by Magherini also occurred in other Italian cities such as Venice and Ravenna. Moreover, in Jerusalem, in the 1990s, psychiatrists and psychologists at the Kfar Shaul Hospital (1991 Bar-El,I) carried out a study analogous to that of Florence and described a clinical condition they called the Jerusalem syndrome, linked to spiritual effects affecting a tourist or an inhabitant of that city. The episode has the form of a psychosis and manifests itself with signs of delirium: the affected person massively identifies with a figure from the history of the Old or New Testament and acts as such, for example, Moses or King David or Jesus of Nazareth or John the Baptist. This identification is usually with persons of the same sex.

Although Magherini places these manifestations within psychopathology, certain issues observed in varying degrees appear in the aesthetic experience described in this book: brief episodes, flashes of bewilderment that cause a kind of blindness unleashed by an intense aesthetic experience. It is possible to trace in the narrative of the protagonists a condensation of sensations, raw intuitions, but also a certain willingness to move in the direction of experience.

4.2 Narcissism, the body and the image and disengagement through art

The concept of narcissism, from the moment Freud—in 1914—introduced it in one of his most complex articles, has been an articulator and parenthesis in Freudian thought. Taken up and deployed by contemporary psycho-analysis in its European and American aspects, it develops ideas on primary and secondary narcissism, original narcissism, life and death narcissism, narcissism as a structure or a state, or a representation of narcissistic charges, understood from the *self*. These theorizations show that it is a concept not susceptible to unification.

We can think of narcissism as pure refraction of the image, nonetheless crossed by the experience of the body, where it is evident that *we are irremediably constituted by the gaze of the other*. The other that confirms us and guarantees us life in early helplessness and thereby attaches us to a *scopic attraction* that anticipates the understanding of the implications of the gaze of others. This constitutive gaze, which shapes us and virtually delimits us—at a time when we experience ourselves as a fragmented disarticulation—, is our fate, and our *lack,* as Lacan postulates in the "mirror stage" and, as Lacan affirms; something always remains outside, below or behind the projected image—in the play of mirrors—, depending on the *position of* the observer. That image is not only loaded with ideal and projection; it will also be transformed by the desire of the Other and by the drive itself, as on a Moebius band[1]. This *configuring gaze makes the uncontrolled bodily "experience", in front of the mirror, an "Aha erlebniz!",*[2] *an* expression of jubilation before the reflected image of the body. *This gaze will act as an erotic mediation that enables the expression of joyful identification, covering it lovingly with a seal that, beyond the word, will impose a meaning.*

This constitutive inadequacy between what we see and what looks at us (Didi-Huberman, 1997), responds to the same dynamics of the phenomenon of art, when the aesthetic experience takes place. As an effect of the image in art and intoxicated by that "soft narcosis" that it provokes, we are dragged towards a particular experience from which the experience itself then rescues us. It is the aesthetic experience that, as a *paradoxical meeting point,* as *mediation, involves* the spectator and the work and establishes a condition of possibility by promoting an *effect of subjectivation.* It is subjectivation because it salvages the questioning of the self from "pure self-referential consciousness" which, when involved by the work, accounts for alienation. The object of artistic creation, for Green (1995, p. 50), narcissistically invested, serves as an object of projection and, nevertheless, also "serves as mediation with the other who enjoys by identification". This identification with the image, with the object, whose predecessor is mimesis, *is a more complex process,* where alienation and objectification, estrangement and appropriation take place, engaging a potentially transforming effect that *goes beyond the idea of identification.* The very image of the aesthetic experience, by "capturing" us and then expelling us from that *place*—in which, let us clarify, one can only remain for an instant—introduces the double quality of alienating and objectifying. It alienates, absorbs and compromises in a carnal identification and, at the same time, as in a movement of return, it dis-alienates and separates by showing us that reality is *other* than that which re-presents the image by which we were *attracted.* This operation, in which the *aesthetic experience* subsumes us, implies a sort of splitting, a splitting of the ego, outside of pathology. As happened to Freud on the Acropolis, a *non-pathological estrangement, a* necessary condition in the encounter with art, promotes a different form of decapsulation of the libido overturning the ego of narcissism *by imposing participation with the object, with Other.* "The act of estrangement in that objectification that every work of art produces is corrective," says Adorno (2004), definitive.

Following this line of argument, we see that in art—as in falling in love, and also in analysis—a leap outward from the self, from one's own body, is favored when the libido, attracted by the "image of the body in art", recovers the lost object *by means of a detour, as a transferred "other"*. The image, *entrapping the gaze,* seduces us as evocation and this seduction of the gaze holds *an invitation*: *a promise*, a promise of pleasure, which in the manner of *previous pleasure* (Freud, 1905) is the pleasure summoned by images that possess maximum attractiveness (*reisz*), not only for aesthetic reasons, but also certain conditions to provoke the interest of Eros. In the aesthetic experience, something of the forbidden, lost object is veiled and revealed, which fulfills this condition of ideal love, a condition of infantile love: to return to *that state* which has always been longed for. But art says something more. First it invites us, seduces us and absorbs us in an experience that we could think of as sensorial ... then it forces us outside ourselves, even beyond what is reflected and also beyond the senses, towards a symbolized representation that introduces a certain narrative, illogical, dislocated. We could say that it is a non-discursive letter: displacement and condensation of a figurative charge. This type of non-discursive language manifests itself as a form of sensibility and conceptuality that constitutes the phenomenon of aesthetic experience.

In Pollock, it is the plastic transmutation of the body in action; in Botticelli, it is the magical evocation of the symbolism hidden in the Greek nymph and in the search for "the natural" of romantic art. An opportunity where "works of art emerge from the empirical world and produce a world with an essence of its own, opposed to the empirical, as if this other world also existed," as Adorno (2004, p. 10) argues. He goes on to say: "In every genuine work of art something appears that does not exist" (p. 113), whereby an *inadequacy* is established, where the *shock* of identification with that which, in reality, is not and the discrimination of that formal identity impose otherness and the decapsulation of narcissism. Then, it is the object, "transformed" in art, between the self and the other, which installs a difference that touches the Other, the beautiful transfigured. Something lost is salvaged and the distant pleasure, which reappears with symbolic efficacy, eroticized.

Narcissism is, according to Green (1998, p. 11), "the cement that keeps the unity of the self-constituted, that has brought together its components, giving it a *formal identity* that is [...] *precious for its feeling of existence*". Therefore, this "cement" comes to constitute a *narcissistic shell.* I understand that art offers a specific condition of possibility for the decapsulation of this shell; because, in each encounter in the aesthetic experience, it is inaugurated, in a desired and feared reencounter, and *in the notion of difference* between the dreamed and devised ideal and what appears in the image: what it is *possible* to represent. As in some works of art, these are reflected in the two forces at play; when the beautiful threatens by an idealized perfection *that appeals to the ominous,* for example, in the dazzling radiance of Moreau's painting, in some perverse glow in Balthus, in Schiele, or in Lucian Freud's painting.

From these references it can be affirmed then that in estrangement forms of pleasure and Eros, a sensuality awakened in that state *activates in the receiver the movements that also took part in the artist during the creative process. These internal movements come from mythical, prehistoric times, and have the evocative force of the senses, of the bodily, of the lost "original"... and of the natural (not to say: the "real"). This enchantment transcends aesthetic pleasure, because it offers something new.* Between sexuality and narcissism, between ego and object libido, through the experience of art the libido is outsourced, the shell is *cracked* through the effect of art. In estrangement, otherness operates in a mediated way, similar to what happens in work in transference inherent to the analytical field. These are the "supreme effects of art" that Freud never ceases to question, which imposes its *function of not knowing* and throws us, in a *moderate way*, towards an anticipated alterity. This is the effect that, like the *mise-en-scène in transference*, eludes the real presence of the other and summons *another real one* that is repressed or rejected. In this act, a process is outsourced which, by penetrating the shell of our petrified bourgeois ego, projects us towards the work, which thus promotes the decapsulation of narcissism ... *an old and new psychic act.*

4.3 Melancholy, iconology and the failed aestheticization of the self

4.3.1 Vincent's two melancholies

There are many ways of thinking about the fate of estrangement in melancholy and art. In the developments of the field of Art History, we find contributions on a melancholy that was also associated with deep, stark introspection about human life; some authors valued it as the engine of philosophical reflection (CITAS) or the propitiation of religious contemplation; These creative faces of melancholy are the artists. Lacan affirms that in creation, the form of the work: art, resists the melancholic temptation of silence and destruction, "resists the death drive"; that is to say, it borders on the real while conserving its tension so that the work lives, as we saw in Trias (2001).

For example, Dürer's Melancholy I, represents a nocturnal, gloomy, cold and solitary environment: a character seated on a stone bench—a woman with angel's wings—, in a meditative state, lost in thought and apparently absent—her enormous eyes open and fixed, with a somber, sad expression, leaning on the closed fist of her left hand, which rests on a closed book, with an enormous compass. On the wall an hourglass, a bell, a seven stepped ladder leaning against the wall. On the floor, carpentry and architectural tools: an inkwell, a pen and two geometric objects -a lathed wooden sphere and a perfectly carved stone polyhedron. On one side we see the shadow cast by the moon on the objects and on the other, the glow of a comet that, as a symbol of evil, is enclosed in a lunar rainbow that projects a strange

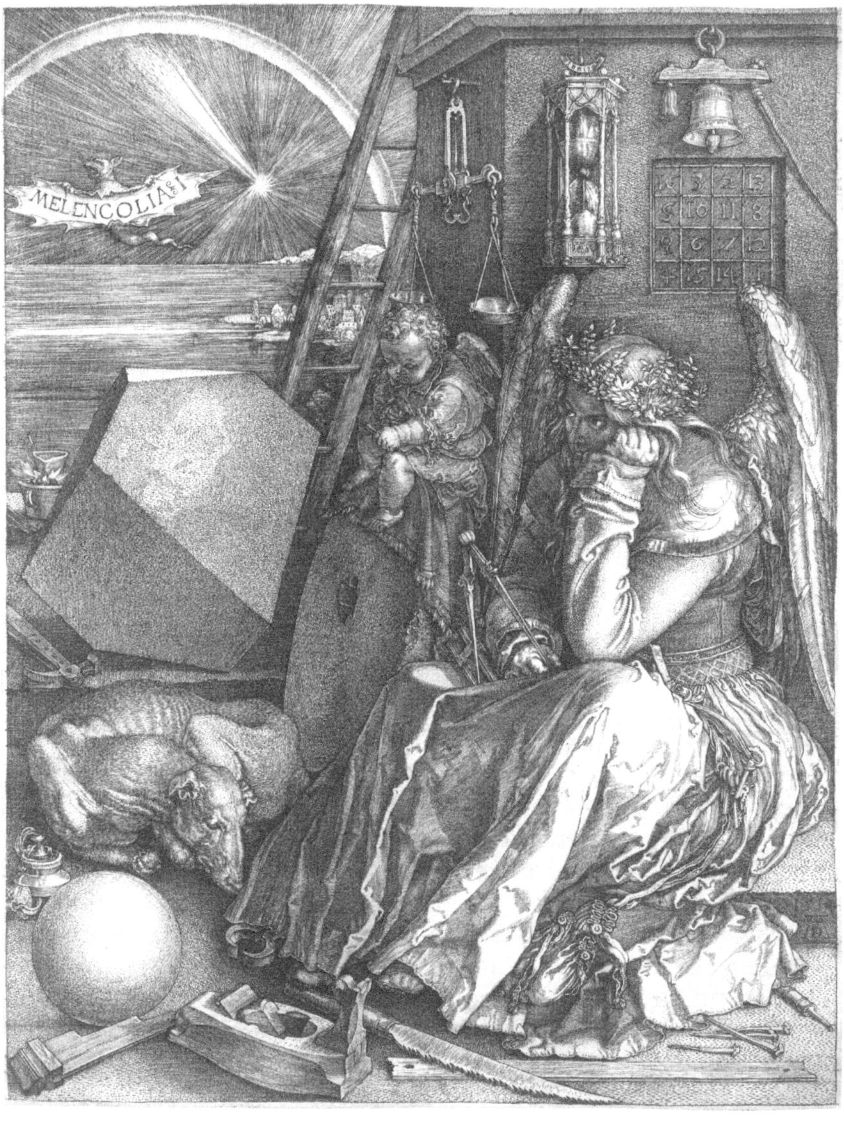

Figure 4.1 Engraving "Melencolia I" (Dürer, A. 1514).

light illuminating the title of the engraving—**MELENCOLIA I**—on a sign bearing a bat (See Figure 4.1).

The complex whole of Dürer's engraving is dominated by the idea of the concentration of the Human Being as a thinking subject who faces the becoming of his existence, who has to seclude himself in an intellectual retreat to reach the light of wisdom and who has the capacity for Art through his melancholic imagination. "Melancholy" is the personification of the intellectual virtue of the secular genius in the rational and imaginary world of science and art. It also represents the artist, who possesses the knowledge and technique to create, but whose inspiration sometimes resists taking flight, although he has the wings that adorn his back, a symbol of imagination and creativity and a manifestation of his intellectual superiority

This relation between art and melancholy has many antecedents; for example, during the Renaissance melancholy was associated with artistic temperament, imagination, and creativity, according to the ideas expressed by Agrippa of Nettesheim in "De Occulta Philosophia", an esoteric text published in 1531, which describes three types of melancholy: "imaginative melancholy", "mental melancholy" and "rational melancholy" (Goldstein, 2005). The first is the one that affects artists; this explains the I of the title of the engraving, MELANCOLIA I, representing the imaginative character of artists. We can work on the artist's exercise when representing, conjuring and giving form to everything that is not himself, which contains so much of the unconscious and of reality. This act of micro-hope highlights the present contemporary psychoanalytic reflection that we are doing today; and the place of art, creativity and their transforming function.

Another emblematic statement is that of Vincent van Gogh. In his letters, references to a profoundly melancholic state are recurrent as a kind of background condition of his life; at the same time, a desperate will to exist appears. In van Gogh, this involves a "lucid distinction of two times of melancholy" following letter to Teo in Recalcati (2019). Abandonment and death, nostalgia, and hopelessness prevail in one. In the other, which he himself defines as "active melancholy," there is energy, vitality. Active melancholy is the singular effort to resist the call to sink into melancholia. Art acquires for van Gogh the features of an active melancholy. How to overcome and counteract melancholia with "positive work"? Its mode of constitution in which the Other assigns him the position of a discarded object nevertheless enables the other, the creative one, the one of Evangelical preaching, to occupy that active Christianity: that is to say, another reflexive in "active melancholy". *The aesthetic experience is a condition of possibility of creativity, the key to working through the mourning and opening up to the understanding of time in the cure.*

In Van Gogh, melancholy and creation go hand in hand; the artist creates in order to create his name and not be trapped in his original melancholy that exposes him to sinking. The stigma of his original melancholy is an indelible identification with the lost thing, the ideal that bears his name like the dead little brother, "denying him symbolic inscription in the field of the other" (Recalcati et al., 2006). This original melancholy that accompanies him all his life due to this identification that has not been permeated by the other's desire is sustained by something lost, because it is dead. Unattainable as an ideal, it tends to produce a melancholic type of identification. The shadow of little Vincent falls over this fire, this substitute child. The parents' desire did not enable the work of mourning. For this reason, Freud insists that additional time is needed. In psychoanalysis, the melancholic position is characterized by a disconnection from the real body, from its narcissistic image, which is not linked to the body because the shadow of the lost object,—his dead little brother (ideal)—falls upon the subject who is unable to inscribe himself in the Other's desire. However, in art there is a time that makes it possible.

Notes

1 N. A: A continuous ribbon that, joined in a twist, does not allow to speak of interior or exterior. It is a product of the 18th century mathematician and astronomer August Ferdinand Moebius.
2 N. A: Expression of "identificatory jubilation" that Lacan attributes to the "mirror stage".

References

Adorno, Th. W. (1970/2004) Teoría estética, Madrid, Ediciones Akal.
Didi-Huberman, G. (1997) Lo que vemos, lo que nos mira, Barcelona, Manantial.
Freud, S. (1905) Fragment of an Analysis of a Case of Hysteria (1905 [1901]). The Standard Edition of the Complete Psychological Works of Sigmund Freud 7: 1–122.
Green, A. (1995) La metapsicologia revisitada, Buenos Aires, Editorial Eudeba.
Green, A. (1998) Las cadenas de Eros, Buenos Aires, Amorrortu Editores.
Goldstein, G. (2005) La experiencia estética, Buenos Aires, del estante editorial.
Magherini, G., (1990) El Síndrome de Stendhal, Madrid, Espasa Calpe-Espasa Mañana, p. 171.
Recalcati, M. (2019) Melancholia y creacion en Vincen van Gogh, España, Nuevos Emprendimientos Editoriales.
Recalcati, M., Brousse, M-H, Wajcman, G., Coccoz, V, Giner Ponce, X, Vinciperra, R.-P. (2006) Las tres estéticas de Lacan, Buenos Aires, Ediciones El Cifrado.
Stendhal, (2017) "El síndrome del viajero", Diario de Florencia, Madrid, Gadir Editorial, pp. 17–22.
Trías, E. (2001) Lo bello y lo siniestro, Barcelona, Ed. Ariel.

5 Estrangement and Creativity, the Cure at Stake

5.1 Strangeness and the edges of the creative processes

In any work of art, in any of its expressions, the archaic and the creative converge, but the work of art, as a creation, is also a re-creation; it not only refers to the past, but also, through symbolism, salvages it and incorporates it into cultural heritage. In this way, the triad past-present-future remains inseparable and in constant interaction, as Ayensa explains (2006). This author places imaginative and perceptual phenomena in the knot of temporal articulation, as well as the coexistence between the conscious and the unconscious that come into play when perceiving.

Authors such as Gaston Bachelard affirm the primitive, psychically fundamental character of creative imagination. Imagination is the basis of all creativity; it is reproductive and productive. Productive imagination has prospective activity, understood as "an adventure of perception" (Bachelard, 1994), and thereby differentiates the perceived image from the created image as two very different psychic instances.

Ayensa (2006) points out:

> Like Bachelard, Gilbert Durand considers imagination as an organizing dynamism and therefore a factor of homogeneity in representation. Imagination is a dynamic power that "deforms" the images provided by perception and re-forms sensations, becoming the foundation of psychic life. Piaget also finds a "functional coherence" between symbolic thought and conceptual sense, which constitutes a unity of the forms of representation. (Ayensa, 2006, p. 239)

It is in this dynamic encounter between imagination and perception that the singular coordinates of representation unfold. This encounter is full of difficulties insofar as this coherence is not achieved within the framework of the aesthetic experience in a plain and direct way, but quite the contrary. It is in the failure of this intention to grant perceptual coherence where the encounter with the ominous is experienced, provoking that state of estrangement, knot of the aesthetic experience.

DOI: 10.4324/9781003591559-6

In estrangement, in that instant of occurrence, something similar to certain "unusual phenomena" happens which, as already mentioned, produce an estrangement regarding the perception of the self or of the object. Freud analyzes them as the momentary admission of a fragment of truth introduced into the conscious in the manner of mental mirages in which we want to recognize something as belonging to our ego or, in alienations, we want to exclude it. In turn, in the case of aesthetic experience, it does its job. As I state in another work: "A fragment of something hidden thus comes to light, and the split and projected no longer returns as strange, since the experience that allows us to see again that which was not well endured before is admitted. And the instant of truth is revealed, threading fantasies, between daydreams and forgotten memories" (Goldstein, 2005, p. 816).

In fact, Freud argues that daydreaming proceeds in the same way as the dream, using the present time for the representational content "It should also be remembered here that it is not only in dreams that such transformations of ideas into sensory images occur: they are also found in hallucinations and visions, which may appear as independent entities, so to say, in health or as symptoms in the psychoneuroses" (Freud P. 535 (S.E.)).

In the field of aesthetic experience, the progredient and the regressive sense are superimposed, in a tilting movement. The dream is not the aesthetic experience, but aspects of the dynamics of the dream are inexorable and present in it. As in psychoanalysis, in the aesthetic experience an inexorable thirdness leads us to a type of process that is part of the experience that produces a new elaboration of the primary and secondary processes.

In this instant, in that present of the aesthetic experience, there is an acceleration of images that unfold—superimposed—as in the paradoxical time of dreams and daydreams. This temporal simultaneity in the aesthetic experience imposes on the observer an encounter with something dislodged, admitting, paradoxically, consciousness and the flow of the unconscious in the same time (outside of pathology).

This encounter takes place in a between-space, in a transitional place of creation, in this movement characterized by a sublimated mode of detachment of pleasure; in the sequence Eros-binding-aesthetic experience, it reveals some mediatized and intertwined processes, in the manner of the processes we call "tertiary" along with Green and others.

In turn, from the new interrelation that these tertiary processes involve a better worked through production results, in the sense of drive, sublimated in the presence of the thirdness characteristic of cultural phenomena and aesthetic experiences.

For Piera Aulagnier (1977), the object exists psychically by virtue of its power to modify the sensory response and thus acts on the psychic experience. It is therefore possible to conceive a model of psyche that is relatively open to the new and the different, as well as to remodeling and neo configurations. Representing (metabolizing) does not imply a flat image of the psyche but rather a complex figure with various facets and dimensions, with depth, perspective, volume, thickness and history. In this sense, the creative deployment, poetic in the sense of production of the psyche, interacts with an object that promotes it; therefore, the work of art invokes the potential of new inscriptions in the representational range.

In another direction, André Green (1995) theorizes on tertiary processes located on the borderline between the Freudian primary and secondary processes. Green's conceptual contribution—undoubtedly a tributary of the *transitional phenomena* described by Winnicott—goes beyond the Freudian analytic goal of turning irrational and unconscious primary processes into rational and conscious secondary processes. Green argues that psychoanalysis seeks to develop the *tertiary*—or intermediary—*processes* that facilitate a fluid, elaborative back and forth between primary and secondary processes. For this author, the possibility of *working through* depends on the way the tertiary processes operate or not, as a way of making the representational field more flexible and allowing the emergence of the new in psychic terms. Green defines them as processes "that put primary and secondary processes in relation in such a way that the primary ones limit the saturation of the secondary ones and the secondary ones of the primary ones", establishing an unstable equilibrium between what is "incessantly shifting" and what is "definitely coagulated".

In this sense, he affirms that the potential exit from the linear duality of a one-to-one relationship (subject-object) implies the mobility of registers and the activation of tertiary processes. This double register (intrapsychic and intersubjective) of the phenomena of encounter favors a "third thought" that emerges from operations of reunion and separation (intersubjective), articulated with the various modes of thought (intrapsychic) "opening a possibility of leaving the impasses of duality"; where the opening to reflexive processes outside duality promotes the emergence of new psychic contents.

In relation to the creative, poietic, tertiary processes, it is Héctor Fiorini (2006) who maintains that:

> The creative processes establish a certain type of temporality, inherent to these processes, which is not reduced to the forms of temporality itself, to the "primary" and "secondary" processes. Neither is it only the temporality of linear time, nor only the temporality of the Freudian unconscious, nor only the retroactivity of certain phenomena studied in psychopathology.
>
> (p. 1)

Fiorini salvages in his theorization on the creative psyche a differential condition to the Freudian approach to works of art, affirming that beyond what the works of art represent, it is a matter of approaching what they *present* as a potentiality of new inscriptions. The crux of his assertions involves defining the psyche insofar as the creator establishes three great places and two limits between those places. In other words, it is a five-element topic.

He maintains:

> ...The creative processes have their starting point there, because no one creates from nothing but from a certain world, a certain horizon, certain already constituted objects... The given challenges the creative psyche to find, in the manner of a Hegelian antithesis, alternatives to the given, to find in the not yet given something that presents alternatives to the already given. Alternatives that have the character of unpublished, unknown or unpredictable.
>
> (Fiorini, 2006, p. 4)

In this way, the already given, the instituted, threatens the psyche with entrapment and, at the same time, the creative psyche pushes against this capturing threat. This drive impels it to cross the limit of what is already given. It is the drive that disorganizes pre-established forms in order to promote new spaces toward the unknown.

In this conflict, in the interior of the psyche, the crossing of a limit occurs, a transgression that entails anxiety and pleasure. Pleasure in terms of freedom, anxiety for the chaos generated in the disorganization. Thus, the moment of creation implies a state of vertigo, of abyss, fascinating, anguishing, at constant risk of blockages and inhibitions, which must give rise to reorganizations in order not to block the creative process. Along the same lines, Rojas (2002) states:

> Creation takes place in two spaces... The space of creation, the uncertain space of origin, is described as a 'sea of possibilities' before which the subject suffers from impotence. For this reason, he has to move towards the second space, where sensitive experience is formed, always ready to go beyond what is known in order to create another language in which expression is equivalent to experience.
>
> (p. 2)

This last statement connects the notion of creative processes with that of *poiesis*, the state of production, as opposed to praxis.

It is worth remembering that Winnicott maintains that in the creative encounter of the analysis a game will be played that will involve not only pointing out repetitions but also developing creativity as a result of the intersubjective involvement of each of the members of the analytic couple with their own primary and secondary processes; thus unfolding the area of illusion in that intermediate and paradoxical field. In the aesthetic experience, the encounter, the friction of the unconscious, allows the unfolding of these creative processes in a transitional and paradoxical space and time.

For Zukerfeld (2002), these creative processes are understood as tertiary processes that allude to the encounter with the split unconscious as creative potential. Encounter and recovery of that which is not represented, never repressed but inaccessible to the conscious, that is made available to the subject in the occurrence of a psychic event, of an instant, of a disruption in the continuity of the psychic process.

He thereby agrees with Rosolato (1978), who differentiates different aspects of the negative, and among them locates the unknowable as that which exists irreducibly and cannot be abolished constituting the limit of all knowledge, like Freud said with an irreducible potential of unknowability.

It thus proposes the intimate relation in the construction of the psyche between soma and the significant other that fulfills the Freudian functions of support and model, where splitting is a foundational mechanism and not only a defense mechanism. This theoretical argumentation finds coincidences with two central aspects that we propose: on the one hand, the creative opportunity that opens up in the encounter of the subject with the object of art—aesthetic experience-; on the other hand, the binding and phenomenic emergence of the state of estrangement from the sensory field, sustained in the soma, in the evident plane of sensations that include a form of sensitive thought.

Up to this point, we have outlined the central notions of the fundamental authors within the psychoanalytic, psychodynamic and aesthetic fields, which enable us to establish the conceptual coordinates necessary to theoretically understand the state of estrangement as a node of the aesthetic experience.

As may be inferred, describing and theorizing about it implies the possibility of conceiving a creative psyche, open to an innovative potential, which emerges in contact with the unconscious and is inaugurated in an instant -shock- of encounter, in a paradoxical space, through this state of estrangement. All these conditions determine the journey through an aesthetic experience, delimited to the field of the encounter with art, but relevant to the psychoanalytic clinical field, since it configures an opportunity for the gestation of psychic change processes.

5.2 The ominous in art and the place of Eros

The *Dictionary of the Royal Spanish Academy* defines "ominous" as follows: "(from *ominosus*) Azaroso, de mal agüero, abominable, vitando." And "vitando": "To be avoided. Hateful, execrable." While ominous is described as a noun, we can also think of it as an adjective that qualifies sensations produced by situations.

Valls (1995) says in his *Freudian Dictionary* about the Ominous:

> There are ominous situations and sensations produced in the subject by them. The sensation of the ominous is a special type of distressing sensation, with its own qualitative characteristics belonging to the order of terror and horror; it is produced by some typical experienced situations, fantasies about them or derived from them. To these characteristic representations, psychoanalysis attributes the origin of this form of unpleasurable affect, qualitatively different and with specific characteristics...
>
> (p. 579).

It is Trías (2001) who, as we quoted above, affirms that "the ominous constitutes the condition and limit of the beautiful". Therefore, "aesthetic effect" cannot occur without being linked to the ominous present in the work. As a limit, the revelation of the ominous is incompatible with the aesthetic effect, thus constituting its condition. Consequently, the ominous is a condition and a limit: it must be present in the form of absence, it must be veiled, it cannot be revealed.

According to Félix Duque, the notion of "the sublime" appears in the first century, in *Pseudo-Longinus*. Heirs of Kantian aesthetics and the feeling of the sublime (*das Erhabene*), a series of philosophers and thinkers such as Hegel, Krause and Schelling assume the Kantian presuppositions and understand beauty as divine presence, incarnation of the infinite in the finite. The feeling of the sublime breaks "the consideration of aesthetics as a theory of the beautiful, forcing it to admit the inhospitable guest (*unheimlich*) of the sublime". But it is Schelling who formulates the definition taken by Freud for his later analysis: "*Unheimlich* is everything that, while it should remain secret, hidden... nevertheless, has manifested itself".

Freud, in his writing "The Uncanny" (1919), comes to the conclusion that *unheimlich* is "something that was always familiar to psychic life and that only became strange through the process of its repression" (p. 28) but for this he begins by pointing out the singularity that the term *unheimlich* itself entails. *Unheimlich* is the antonym of *heimlich*, that which is familiar, Freud points out, from which it follows "obviously" that the *Unheimlich* would be that "which causes fright precisely because it is known, familiar" (p. 12); but the problem lies in the fact that not everything that is new causes fright, nor everything that is familiar is "immunized" against the ominous. Moreover, *heimlich* is not always an antonym of *unheimlich*, but rather the opposite.

Continuing with Freud's study, the notion of *Unheimlich* should be understood as that which, through the process of its repression—as a rejection of ideas or desires that may be considered harmful to the subject—shows a hidden and inhospitable face in the familiar by making visible that which consciousness would prefer to have forgotten ... And what is more familiar than language itself? What is more forgotten than its own origin, always latent and at the same time, always present?

From the Freudian perspective, those desires seeking fulfillment and discharge, due to their repulsive character, must constantly be forced to remain unconscious. This unconscious dynamic is generated by repression, the action by which unacceptable thoughts are actively and energetically prevented from entering consciousness. Trying to come to light, the strength of that which is repressed lies precisely in its hidden character. In this sense *Unheimlich* and *Heimlich* mean the same thing: the mysterious, the hidden, the secret. "So *heimlich* is a voice whose meaning evolves into ambivalence until it ends up coinciding with that of its antithesis, unheimlich" (p. 28), says Freud. *Unheimlich* is, in short, something familiar that has become strange and inhospitable or, in the words of Eugenio Trias (2001): "*something that, upon revealing itself, shows itself in its ominous face, despite being, or precisely because it is, in reality, in depth, very familiar, the most inherently familiar, intimate, recognizable*" (p. 42).

The question, however, is not yet resolved, Freud points out, since even admitting that the ominous is that which has been repressed and has returned from repression, it cannot be affirmed that everything that alludes to those repressed desires is ominous. To resolve this difficulty in his approach, Freud distinguishes between the experienced or not experienced ominous and the imagined or fictional ominous. The experienced ominous, which occurs less frequently and depends on much simpler conditions, can emerge in primitive ways of thinking that come to light before any event that could confirm them and in which the material reality of the former is raised (for example, the return of death or the phenomenon of the double); or from repressed infantile complexes, in which the question of material reality is not even raised, appearing instead, the psychic reality. Here the ominous refers specifically to the repression of its psychic content and the return of the repressed.

The ominous in art, in fantasy (or in the artistic work), on the other hand, manifests itself in a more complex way. As Freud argues in "The Uncanny", certain frightening objects or fantasies refer not directly to terror but to unbridled desires. These objects of art that manage to promote the link with that lost object, manage to capture the spectator, enrapture him, deceive him and, in that encounter, on that edge, something of one's own, experienced as alien, slips in. Something of the repressed, of the unremembered, a trace of that primordial experience becomes a sensation and awakens the alien quality of memory.

It is evident how the description of the characteristics of the state of estrangement, from a psychoanalytic perspective, consolidates a somewhat circular conceptual articulation of interdependent terms that interdefine each other, where each is a condition of the other. The framework is the possible relation between art and psychoanalysis, where the meeting point lies in the understanding and theorization of the unconscious processes involved both in artistic creation and in the occurrence of an aesthetic experience.

In the experience with art, a new paradigm emerges in which Eros reappears in the conflict intrinsic to its nature. As I state in *The Aesthetic Experience*: "Let us remember that Eros, for the Greeks, is the representative not only of erotic love but of all creative impulse, he emerges—according to the Theogony—, after the initial chaos together with Gaia and the underworld" (Goldstein, 2005). The mythological Eros shows, from its origin, the contradiction that constitutes it, as happens with Freud's Eros, which is at the same time conflict and cohesive force. Art as an encounter with the beautiful, at the same time, approaches the sublime, the ominous. The difference imposed by art and the encounter with art as an aesthetic experience is a form of pleasure that is a promise of pleasure, "Promise of happiness", as Stendhal would say, that looks to the disturbing, but is sustained within a symbolic "frame".

5.3 The bonds of Eros

Freud states in the final sentence of *The Ego and the Id* in 1923: "... we are concerned that we thus underestimate the role of Eros". The aesthetic experience is an encounter with art that as an event involves a disruptive effect and a feeling of estrangement, which promotes a paradoxical pleasure. We cannot underestimate the role of Eros which, in this complex of sensations and reasons, appears in the form of a lost, nostalgic or disturbing object, diverse modes of pleasure emerge, which we call paradoxical pleasure. There is no aesthetic experience in which pleasure is not involved, since art is a "promise of happiness", a promise that, according to Stendhal, announces the encounter with the beautiful, the desired, in terms of art, a promise that he equates to that produced by love. Both love and art are a promise, a promise of happiness, a promise of pleasure. Beyond the fact that for Freud, the program of happiness is unrealizable and that for Adorno the promise of happiness is a broken promise, it is precisely because of this that the aesthetic experience, as a paradoxical pleasure, is also something of happiness that, in its impossibility, involves thinking, feeling and thinking, a new way of thinking that includes lost affects or, what is possible in a new experience of pleasure, that traces other coordinates.

Eros, as pleasure, is necessarily involved and is what accompanies as the most open modes of bonding that connect the lost, the foreign, the alien of one's own and the strangeness of the world. Eros as binding, re-launches its bonds by threading something of the unknown, which is confronted in the object of art as an object of the world of culture. The phenomena of the aesthetic experience, beyond the sublime or ominous of the strange encounter, are, as long as they are not pathological, strangeness with the predominance of Eros.

The Eros of art appears linked to paradoxical pleasure and may sometimes refer to a type of pleasure that runs through the whole body, more directly in relation to what Freud considers the archetype of bliss that comes from sexual love in its origin, since "… one of the forms of manifestation of love, sexual love, has given us the most intense experience of overwhelming pleasurable sensation, thus giving us the archetype for our aspiration to bliss", says Freud in "civilization and it discontents" (1930, p. 81). That pleasure is facilitated by the conditions in which the aesthetic experience takes place, given that in estrangement, ties with reality are loosened in the midst of a kind "narcosis", in that particular encounter, this space is, as Juan Ritvo said in the quote above, "the site par excellence of experience in moments of slumber, of relaxation of links, of suffering, of orgasm …" and is related to reflection, rapture and also mind clouding. In this way, something surpasses the level of sensory localization, of the visual, generating effect: an "orgasmic" effect.

It is worth arguing, following Freud's idea of the "oceanic feeling", a subject for a different research project; it is understood that in the sexual and paradoxical root that includes the subject by moving his unconscious stratum in this form of pleasure, the oceanic feeling may refer to a level of understanding of pleasure, such as "getting lost" or "being missed" or "being captured", a fusional experience outside of pathology, the sexual component radiating its heat, a complex pleasure no longer only buffering part of the experience, but needing the complexity of this paradoxical pleasure found in aesthetic experience. The loosening of the links with the conscious, through aesthetics, as a relaxation of repression and permeabilization of psychic censures, already accounts for a pleasure in itself, which must continue as an aesthetic experience if it succeeds in moving the living, the pathos, the conflict, which touches that of the unconscious nucleus: a resonator in the real that enables the unconscious to emerge in a creative act.

This relief of tensions occurs in a spatial, transitional dimension, in its interplay of inside-outside, I, the Other, intrapsychic and intersubjective, a place of the instant and estrangement that finds a topologic space. It is intermediate space, since these phenomena occur in the space of culture. Winnicott (1971/1998) says: "But the phenomena that possess reality in the zone whose existence I postulate belong to the experience of the relationship with objects" (p. 173). In that place where the creations of human culture may be placed, it is a place conceptualized in Winnicott as "the third zone", a derivative of play. In that zone, there is "relief" from the tension imposed by the "never-ending task of the acceptance of reality, the eternal human task of linking inner and outer reality" (p. 201), writes Winnicott.

Pleasure and Eros, in Freud, are related to happiness in life, which is sought above all in the enjoyment of beauty, both for our senses and our judgment. Although the promise of happiness, as a promise of pleasure, for Freud is unrealizable, he recognizes in art and beauty something of that possibility, although he also says that for the discontent in culture there is no definitive relief. We also see the knot of fantasy released as pleasure in Susana, our interviewee who recounted her experience at the Venice Carnival "as of plenitude or floating ... It's the whole environment. I don't know how to explain it. There was no room for anything else. I was happy" According to Gilbert Rose, it implies the existence of the "necessary illusion".

Illusion, feeling of happiness, and the *sensation of floating or plenitude* manifest one of the necessary modes of Eros that runs through the experiences, something of losing oneself, letting oneself go or floating, is the condition of possibility of aesthetic experience, and modes of pleasure. It is that "the homeland of man is pleasure" insists Agamben, in *Childhood and History*. "In the encounter with art, the image entraps the gaze and produces resonances that make our body vibrate, awakening it to zones of unsuspected sensuality, as happens in Freud's "screen memories" (1899), which "activate an unconscious memory and disguise a forbidden desire". Art makes visible that which is forbidden, that which is impossible to see. When the gaze directed to the work runs through the *whole* work, the totality of *the represented image* ... the aesthetic experience eroticizes an integrating and paradoxical experience. This takes up the idea of aesthetic enjoyment according to Jauss, when he affirms that the attitude of aesthetic enjoyment, in the imaginative conscious, detaches itself from the coercion of customs and interests, thereby freeing the subject from daily chores and enabling him for another experience, producing a "liberation through aesthetic experience and opening to subjectivity insofar as it opens up to intersubjective experience". This movement accounts for the function of play and pleasure as liberation.

Throughout the analysis of the narratives emerging in the interview stories, various adjectives emerged that colored the forms of pleasure felt by the interviewees: references to feelings of happiness, sensuality, eroticism, on the one hand; epiphanic and mystical pleasures linked to immensity, religiosity or eternity, on the other; intense feelings of restlessness, fear, mystery or darkness as well. On very few occasions, the references to the pleasure felt were not paradoxical. The paradox is given, to a certain extent, by the bodily and sensorial anchorage of estrangement. Shock and surprise is felt in the body as excitement and at the same time as tension. The relation with Freudian developments on previous pleasure, pleasure muffled or without discharge, gave an account of this paradoxical modality of feeling pleasure.

On the other hand, as Kant pointed out, pleasure is linked to the sensation of ecstasy or epiphany. It is not possible to separate "the beautiful" from the overwhelming encounter with immensity. In this sense, pleasure is ambiguous, since it expresses a disturbing, ungraspable mode of beauty. That which is unfathomable, vertiginous, refers to the strange, even its own strangeness, which emerges as a somatic mark, felt to be inhospitable and alien.

The *pleasure Ego* summoned up takes us back to distant times when reality remained in suspense and pleasure was dilated, time delayed. Already in the famous letter 52 (December 1896), in the last sentence, Freud speaks of the repetition of the prehistoric unforgettable one. "That unforgettable prehistoric other whom no later one equals anymore," he says in that letter to Fliess: the other of the narcissistic reflex, the other who identifies me. It is a temporary regression, outside of pathology, to "times when the ego had not yet clearly separated itself from the outside world, nor from the Other" (Freud, 1919, p. 236).

These are the times of the inscription of traces, of the mythical experience of satisfaction, when the pleasure ego extends its experience in the instant, incalculable in chronological time. The instant is paradoxical and ungraspable; it joins and divides past and future; according to Agamben (2001), the instant "is always 'other'; this is its nature and is the foundation of the radical 'otherness' of time".

Continuing with Agamben, we see that, in the instant, under certain conditions, a liberating dimension emerges when it articulates, "as an inextensive and ungraspable point," with the "idea of pleasure" as the original human dimension, where time is transformed into history as a liberating instant".

Coinciding with Agamben's (1995) description of the place of aesthetic experience, we say, in the author's words, that it is in that place "situated between narcissistic love and external object choice that the creations of human culture can be placed" ...Winnicott (1971/1998) states: "The place cultural experience is the potential space that exists between the individual and the environment, times of the first experiences that exist there between the subjective object and the object perceived in objective form, between the extensions of the self and the not-self".

The encounter in the aesthetic experience relates to something from which it liberates us. In this respect, André Green argues that the "chains of Eros" unfold according to a series of formations: the drive and its drive motions, the state of pleasure and its correlate, unpleasure and desire expressed as a state of expectation and search, the fantasies, which organize the script of desire, the erotic love language of sublimations.

Eros, in this movement characterized by a sublimated mode of detachment of pleasure and in the sequence Eros-binding-aesthetic experience, reveals some mediatized and intertwined processes, in the manner of processes that we call "tertiary", as I affirm together with Green. We think that, in this creative movement, between illusion and disillusion—poetic in the sense of making and playing and metaphorizing—, it accounts for what Zukerfeld (2002) and Fiorini (2006) call tertiary processes, product of the encounter in relation to the lost object, which appears, in turn, as alien: "It is the lost object as such", says Freud.

It could be said that the aesthetic experience has the character of both an experience in its own right and also a foreign one. Thus, aesthetic experience is the experience in which "man *manages to 'meet the world as at home'* depriving the outside world of its *elusive strangeness*", says Jauss (2002, p. 42). Art, as a place of experience, says Innerarity, "implies that it has produced subject effect, gain, as disinterested pleasure at a point that touches the self and moves it from its certainties or brings something new and incorporates it … the 'human self-understanding' that is culture".

These phenomena produce an opening to subjectivity as an aesthetic experience and highlight the function of play, in the dimension that unfolds the space of culture. Winnicott, in playing and *Reality*, postulates the potential space, a place of psychic constitution, a dimension of illusion, neither reality nor fantasy, but rather a place of intermediation conceptualized as "the third zone", a derivative of play. Freud (1920) writes:

> the artistic play and artistic imitation carried out by adults, which, unlike children's, are aimed at an audience, do not spare the spectators (for instance, in tragedy) the most painful experiences and can yet be felt by them as highly enjoyable. This is convincing proof that, even under the dominance of the pleasure principle, there are ways and means enough of making what is in itself unpleasurable …} into a subject to be recollected and worked over in the mind.
>
> (p. 17)

How is it that in repetition something of pleasure is evoked? Beyond working through and a paradoxical mode of pleasure, there is participation, which means, at the same time, that playing always demands a "playing-with". Gadamer maintains "That is nothing other than *participation,* the inner participation in that movement that repeats itself" (Gadamer, 1993, p. 69). That which inexorably evokes the subject is in that encounter, that "with", with itself and with playing, with the Other. According to the author, the impulse to movement is self-movement that "…indicates a phenomenon of excess of the self-representation of the living being" (Gadamer, 1993, p. 69).

How is it that play as a function of aesthetic experience, free play of imagination and understanding, as Kant puts it, can "unspeakably enlarge the field of what can be thought"? On the other hand, Hegel (1989) maintains that "*Aisthesis* designates the fundamental aesthetic experience in which a work of art can renew the perception of things" which implies conceptual knowledge. From the point of view of reception, its peculiar temporality distinguishes aesthetic experience from other functions of the world of life: it makes us see things anew and provides through this discovering function the enjoyment of a fuller present; it leads to other worlds of fantasy and suppresses the constriction of time; it anticipates future experiences and thereby opens the field of play to possible actions …", says Jauss (2002, p. 71).

As an attempted synthesis, explanations of the paradoxical modes of pleasure produced are knotted: this pleasure is both positive and disturbing at the same time, because the object is ambiguous and refers to a lost object, that awakens nostalgia, that recovers remnants of the subject where the experience of satisfaction and loss left their mark. Touching that unconscious edge, promoted by the encounter in an illusory space with the work of art disarticulates the psychic process from an instant, from a shock that marks a discontinuity in the daily experience. There, time changes its rhythm, and in this state of certain unreality, subjects find themselves and feel. They feel moved in their most intimate part, and tertiary processes emerge that allow them unprecedented creative displays and new meanings.

5.4 The construction of time: The cure at stake

In order to enable the creative potentiality of the instant of each event, the constitution of *an intermediate position* is necessary: the temporary and evanescent union between reality and fantasy as a function of creation. The admission of the beautiful implies its instantaneous quality, so that the ominous appears only as an apparition, as a bias. Therefore, the "overcoming" of trauma is not only a question of change, but *the acceptance of a certain limit* in spite of which meaning is sustained and where, by virtue of the imagination, a temporary and provisional union between sensitivity and comprehension is facilitated in the construction of the lost object. In this particular statute of transitory temporality, the loss and construction of the object is contemplated, administering its extraterritoriality determined by the impulse towards a different logic (approaching paradox). In that time and space, *something* is presented that overflows it and cannot be reduced to concepts. Between the plus and the residue, we can border the system. This perception that seems evanescent is not; it is transcending the immaterial space operated by time in its transitory form, which involves the acceptance of a borderline situation such as symbolic castration; in the aesthetic experience as a transfigured, estranged scene, a new horizon unfolds that, through aesthetic enjoyment, touches the distant unconscious and recovers the time in play of an unfinished history.

References

Agamben, G. (1995) Homo sacer. Il potere sovrano e la nuda vita, Einaudi, Turín.
Agamben, G. (2001) Infancia e historia, Buenos Aires, Adriana Hidalgo Editora.
Aulagnier, P. (1997/1977) La violencia de la interpretación; del pictograma al Enunciado, Buenos Aires, Amorrortu.
Ayensa, A. (2006) In Defense of imagination as the foundation of psychic life and creativity. Logos. Annals of the Seminar on Metaphysics, 39, 235–250.
Bachelard, G. (1994) Water and dreams. Essays on the imagination of matter, Spain, Fondo de Cultura Económica, 1994.

Fiorini, H. (2006) "Formations of tertiary processes. A topic of the creative psyche", in "The Creating Psyche: Theory and Practice of Tertiary Processes" by Hector Juan Fiorini; translated by Susan Rogers. Vitoria-Gasteiz, Spain: Producciones Agruparte. 2006, p.1.
Freud, S. (1919) The 'Uncanny'. The Standard Edition of the Complete Psychological Works of Sigmund Freud 17: 217–256.
Freud, S. (1920) Beyond the Pleasure Principle. The Standard Edition of the Complete Psychological Works of Sigmund Freud 18: 1–64.
Freud, S. (1923) The Ego and the Id. The Standard Edition of the Complete Psychological Works of Sigmund Freud 19: 1–66.
Freud, S. (1930) Civilization and its Discontents. The Standard Edition of the Complete Psychological Works of Sigmund Freud, Volume XXI (1927–1931): The Future of an Illusion, Civilization and its Discontents, and Other Works, 57–146.
Gadamer, H. G. (1993) Verdad y método. Fundamentos de una hermenéutica filosófica, HERMENEIA 7, Quinta Edición. Ediciones Sígueme – Salamanca.
Green, A. (1995) La metapsicologia revisitada", Buenos Aires, Editorial Eudeba
Goldstein, G. (2005) La experiencia estética, Buenos Aires, del estante editorial.
Hegel, G. W. F. (1989) Lessons in Aesthetics. Volume I. Translation from German by Raúl Gabas, Barcelona, Ediciones, p. 62.
Jauss, H. R. (2002) Pequeña apología de la experiencia estética, Barcelona, Paidós, p. 42.
Rojas, J. A. (2002) The work of creation: a creation that works. Implicit theories elaborated by artistic creators. Actualidades en Psicología, 18(105), 70.
Rosolato, G. (1978) La relación de desconocido, Madrid, Ediciones Petrel
Trías, E. (2001) Lo bello y lo siniestro, Barcelona, Ariel.
Valls, J. L. (1995) Diccionario freudiano, Spain, Julián Yébenes, p. 579.
Winnicott, D. (1971/1998) Realidad y juego, Barcelona, Gedisa.
Zukerfeld, R. (2002) "Psicoanálisis, vulnerabilidad somática y resiliencia." IV Congreso Argentino de Psicoanálisis, Rosario, mayo de 2002.

Index

For Product Safety Concerns and Information please contact our
EU representative GPSR@taylorandfrancis.com Taylor & Francis
Verlag GmbH, Kaufingerstraße 24, 80331 München, Germany